Scoliosis

Scoliosis

DIAGNOSIS AND MANAGEMENT

RENE CAILLIET, M.D.

Chairman and Professor
Department of Rehabilitation Medicine
University of Southern California
School of Medicine
Los Angeles, California

F. A. DAVIS COMPANY, Philadelphia

Library of Congress Cataloging in Publication Data

Cailliet, Rene.
  Scoliosis: diagnosis and management.

  Bibliography: p.
  Includes index.
  1. Scoliosis. I. Title. [DNLM: 1. Scoliosis—
Diagnosis. 2. Scoliosis—Therapy. WE735 C134s]
RD771.S3C34   617'.375   75-6709
ISBN 0-8036-1640-6

PREFACE

Scoliosis is the most deforming orthopedic problem confronting children. It is a potentially progressive condition that affects children during their active growth phase and essentially subsides upon completion of spinal growth, leaving the child with a permanent deformity. Early recognition and early treatment can be effective in halting its progress and in many cases result in improvement.

The effects of scoliosis in the child and its persistence into adulthood are primarily cosmetic. However, pain can be significant even after therapy and severe scoliosis can result in cardiopulmonary complications that can decrease life span.

Tremendous strides are being made in the treatment of severe scoliosis, but the desire for early nonoperative treatment is of paramount importance. Only early recognition makes early therapeutic intervention possible.

The purpose of this book is to introduce the subject of scoliosis to all professional and nonprofessional people who come in contact with children. Making them aware of its early manifestations, methods of examination, early treatment, and the more recognized form of surgical treatment will, hopefully, decrease the unnecessarily large percentage of deformed and disabled adults.

Many have helped and supported me in this endeavor. I wish

to give special thanks to Dr. Joel Satzman for his valuable comments, to my colleagues in the Scoliosis Research Society, and to my secretaries, Mrs. Betty Benefield and Mrs. Betty Hemphill, for proofreading and typing my manuscript.

Rene Cailliet, M.D.

Contents

List of Illustrations

CHAPTER 1

Definition
and Natural History
of Scoliosis

Scoliosis, a term of antiquity first used by Hippocrates, implies abnormal curvature of the spine. This skeletal problem is primarily an affliction of children whose spine is growing. There are numerous theories of the etiolology of scoliosis, but the true causative factors remain unknown; thus this affliction currently cannot be prevented. Treatment essentially consists of early recognition, correction of existing curves, and prevention of the further progression of the curves.

The symptoms of scoliosis are primarily those of undersirable appearance with all its physical and psychological components. Since cosmesis is the major sequela of scoliosis, it is unfortunate that idiopathic scoliosis, which is the most prevalent, is present in girls on a ratio of 9:1 compared with boys. Back pain, either in the lumbar or thoracic area, is considered another reason for the treatment of scoliosis. In severe scoliosis, thoracic spine curvature with associated rib cage deformity presents the most serious reason for treating scoliosis. This deformity causes respiratory impairment with possible secondary cardiac complications. These three sequelae (cosmesis, pain, and cardiopulmonary complications) are considered the three reasons why there is the need for early recognition and treatment.

Spinal curvatures of scoliosis progress in a lateral direction

1

and are accompanied by a rotatory deformity pattern. Vertebral body rotation is related to convexity and concavity of the curvature and is greatest at the apical vertebra of the curve. In the thoracic spine, the rib attachment to the vertebrae results in rib cage deformity.

All scoliosis in children with remaining epiphyseal growth must be considered potentially progressive. Progression of scoliosis in the growing spine is the result of vertebral body changes, whereas lesser degree of progression of the scoliosis is possible after cessation of spinal growth because of angular deterioration of the intervertebral disks. This latter incidence of progression is more prevalent in curves of 50° or more.

Treatment of scoliosis over the centuries has included bed rest, traction, symmetrical and asymmetrical exercises, bracing, and surgery. All forms of treatment have had the objective of correcting the cosmetic deformity, preventing further progression and, if present, alleviating pain or cardiorespiratory symptoms. The method of treatment chosen remains relatively arbitrary, although early conservative treatment has gratifying results. Surgical treatment of scoliosis as an orthopaedic problem or advanced case is essentially a salvage procedure or is a more rewarding approach when nonsurgical methods have failed during the early milder conditions.

To date, with no accepted causes known, in most cases prevention or "cure" is not possible. There is now going on international research and exchange of ideas and discoveries that promises significant hope in the search for causes and better treatment methods.

Scoliosis, once considered a rare orthopaedic problem, is now estimated to be present in 1.4 per thousand of the population, with approximately 2 percent of the adult population demonstrating some degree of spinal curvature. Admittedly the "early and mild" cases offer the best prognoses and respond best to conservative treatment. Ultimately it can be hoped that early recognition of all scoliosis will result in decreasing the number of patients who require corrective surgery or, when a significant curve already exists, will initiate early, less extensive, and less radical surgery in order to minimize further progression and its complications. It is in this quest that this monograph is being written: to alert the pediatrician, the family physician, the internist, the physical therapist, the nurse, the physical education teacher, and parents to the value of early recognition. An international education program of early detection and early referral would minimize or prevent the severe deformities and disabilities noted in the adult population.

Many conservative nonoperative procedures have been advocated and their benefits extolled. Many refinements have been made in diagnosis, and surgical procedures have progressed remarkably. Pioneers in scoliosis have not only stimulated their medical colleagues to pursue the search for causative factors but also have stressed to them the desirability of early recognition of the affliction. Space does not permit enumeration of all the physicians who have contributed to scoliosis research.

The intent of this brief monograph is not to be a thorough dissertation on the subject of scoliosis, but to simplify and stimulate knowledge of this condition so that early recognition will result in proper treatment and prompt referral to the orthopaedic specialist whose expertise and interest in scoliosis will initiate proper care.

CHAPTER 2

Normal Spinal Anatomy

The normal spine is composed of 33 vertebrae, separated by intervertebral disks superincumbent on each other, that form the vertebral column (Fig. 1). The entire column, supported upon the sacrum in vertical alignment, forms four physiological curves (Fig. 2). These four curves are termed cervical and lumbar lordosis with the convexity anteriorly and dorsal and sacral kyphosis with convexity posteriorly.

The erect stance is balanced upon an angled sacrum that forms the lumbosacral angle with the horizontal plane. The head must be well balanced above the sacrum so that a plumb line visably passes through the ear, through the shoulder joint, through the greater trochanter of the femur, slightly anterior to the knee joint midline, and ends anterior to the lateral malleolus. These are clinically discernible surface landmarks (Fig. 3). A similar center of gravity when viewed anteriorly-posteriorly should pass from the occiput through the tip of the coccyx.

Stance in the erect position is considered *static* and is termed *posture*. The erect body is intermittently supported by ligamentous tissues and muscles with good erect balance requiring that physiological ligamentous support alternate with minimal isometric muscle contraction. When the spine moves in any direction away from the balanced erect stance, the

5

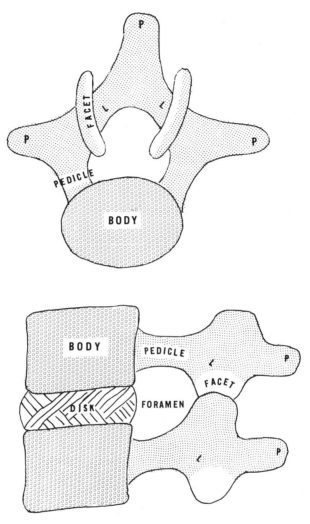

FIGURE 1. Functional Vertebral Unit. The **upper** figure is a view of the vertebral body, the posterior articulations (facets), the pedicles, the processes (**P**), and the lamina (**L**). The lateral view of the unit (**bottom**) demonstrates the intervertebral disk and its relationship to the components of the unit.

direction and extent of movement varies at various segments of the vertebral column. The direction of movement is determined by the plane of the posterior joints (facets), and the extent of motion is limited by the joint capsules, intervertebral disks, ligaments, and muscles.

6

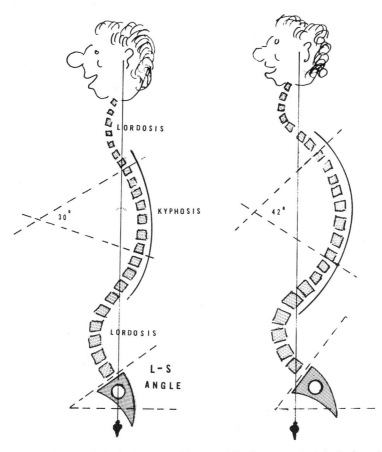

FIGURE 2. Physiological Postural Curves. The figure on the **left** depicts the physiological curves with the head directly above the pelvis. The dorsal kyphosis is approximately 30°, which is physiological. There is also a slight lumbar lordosis. The figure to the **right** shows a "round back" caused by increased dorsal kyphosis. The head is held forward of the center of gravity. The lumbar lordosis is exaggerated because of an increased lumbosacral (**L-S**) angle.

Movement of the lumbar spine is essentially that of flexion-extension with little or no lateral motion or rotation. Forward flexion consists essentially of slight reversal of lordosis with some degree of excessive lordosis possible with hyperextension (Fig. 4). The direction of motion of the lumbar spine is determined by the vertical sagittal plane of the posterior articulations (facets), which are in complete approximation on ex-

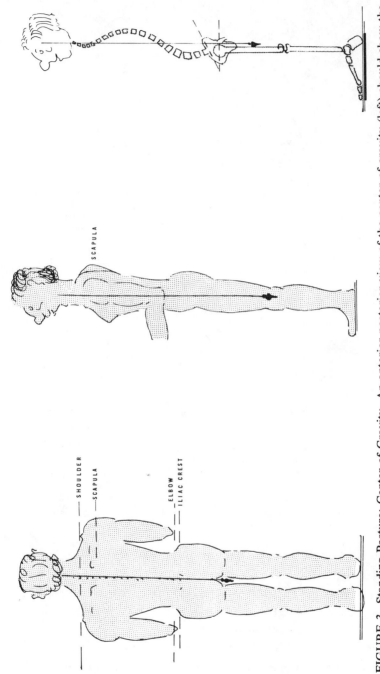

SCAPULA

SHOULDER
SCAPULA

ELBOW
ILIAC CREST

FIGURE 3. Standing Posture: Center of Gravity. An anterior-posterior view of the center of gravity (left) should show the plumb line decending from the occiput through the sacrum. A lateral view (middle and right) should show the plumb line passing through the cervical vertebrae, through the shoulder of the dangling arm, posterior to the hip joint, anterior to the center of the knee joint, and slightly anterior to the ankle lateral malleoli.

8

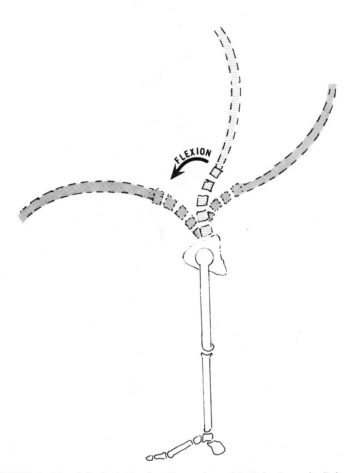

FIGURE 4. Physiological Flexion-Extension of Lumbothoracic Spine. In forward flexion, the thoracic spine flexes an insignificant degree. All flexion occurs in the lumbar spine to the extent of reversal of normal lumbar lordosis. In hyperextension, all motion occurs in the lumbar area with no significant extension occurring in the thoracic region. Most motion of the lumbar spine occurs in the L_4-L_5 and L_5-S_1 region.

tension allowing no lateral or rotatory motion (Fig. 5). Slight forward flexion, which is reversal of lumbar lordosis, permits the posterior facets to separate, thus allowing some lateral and rotatory motion.

The adult thoracic spine has little or no alteration of the physiological kyphosis in forward flexion or extension. The plane of the facets denies this motion but allows lateral rotatory

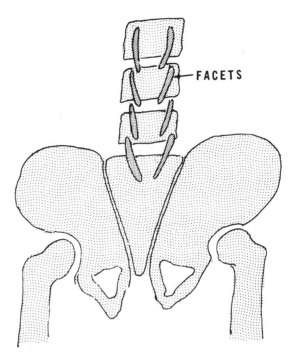

FIGURE 5. Facet Alignment. An anterior-posterior view of the lumbosacral spine shows the plane and alignment of the facets. By their sagittal alignment, they permit flexion and extension of the spine and restrict or limit lateral and rotatory motion.

movement. Thus the vertebral column on lateral and rotatory motion moves essentially in the thoracic area. As the ribs attach and articulate with the thoracic vertebrae, they also exert some limitation of motion and range (Fig. 6). Because of their attachment, when there is abnormal motion or curving of the thoracic vertebrae, as in scoliosis, the ribs are simultaneously curved to assume an abnormal motion and position (Figs. 7 and 8).

The cervical spine has movement from the occiput to the first thoracic vertebra in all directions of flexion, extension, bilateral rotation, or combinations thereof. When viewed laterally the head should be held directly above the plumb-line center of gravity, thus avoiding the "forward head posture" and excessive dorsal kyphosis, or "round back."

10

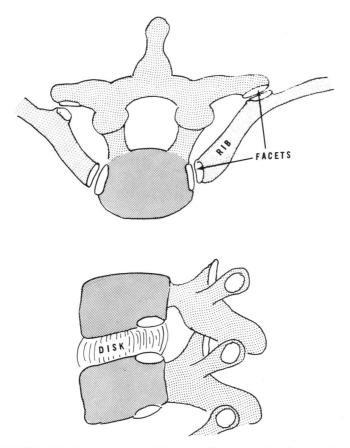

FIGURE 6. Rib Articulations to Thoracic Vertebrae. The head of the rib articulates with two vertebrae to the facets of the vertebral bodies. The tubercle of the rib articulates with the facet at the end of the transverse process. The head of the rib also attaches to the intervertebral disk via an intra-articular ligament. The costotransverse ligament binds the rib to the transverse process.

The intervertebral disks constitute approximately one quarter of the length of the vertebral column and function as hydraulic shock absorbers permitting compression and distortion. In their torsion facility they allow flexion, extension, rotation, or combinations of these motions. The disks are essentially mucopolysaccharide gelatinous tissue consisting of a central mass, the nucleus, contained within an elastic container, the annulus (Fig. 9).

11

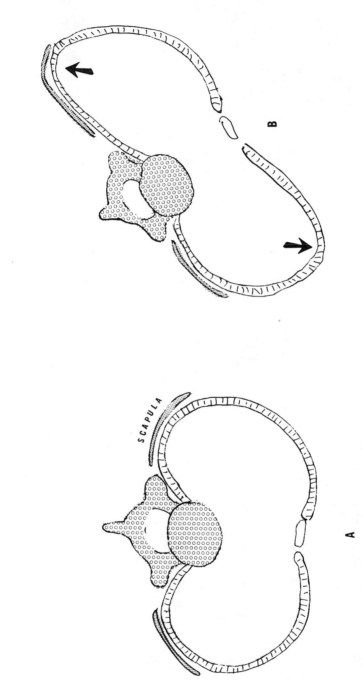

FIGURE 7. Rib Articulations to Thoracic Vertebra. A shows the relationship of the ribs to the vertebral bodies and their contour. B illustrates that since there is rotation of the vertebral body, the rib undergoes deformaton with posterior "humping" (see arrows).

12

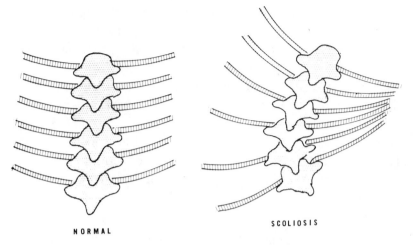

NORMAL

SCOLIOSIS

FIGURE 8. Rib Cage in Scoliosis. In the normal spine the ribs remain parallel and symmetrical. In scoliosis the ribs on the convex side of the curve separate, and those on the concave side approximate.

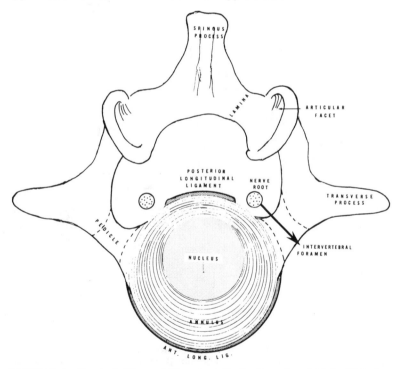

FIGURE 9. Vertical View of Vertebral Body Functional Unit. This is a vertical view of a schematic lumbar vertebra.

The annulus fibers connect around the entire periphery of the vertebral end-plates and intertwine at approximately a 30° angle (Fig. 10). By this arrangement, flexion, extension, and rotation motion is permitted and simultaneously restricted. The nucleus, totally contained within the inner fibers of the annulus and between the opposing vertebral end-plates, is placed under pressure. The intradural pressure of the annulus is approximately one atmosphere (15 kg/cm²) and is partially responsible for the elongation of the vertebral column, its length, its flexibility, and maintenance of the ligamentous tension that supports the column.

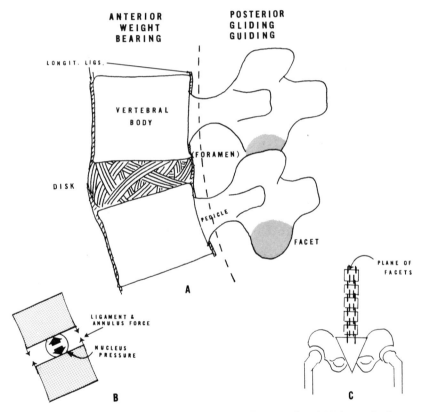

FIGURE 10. Lateral View of Vertebral Body Functional Unit. **A** depicts the lateral view of a lumbar functional unit. **B** shows the interdiskal pressure causing separation of the vertebral bodies. **C** depicts the posterior view of the vertebral column showing the saggital plane of the facets.

14

External pressure exerted upon the disk compresses it, causing deformity and allowing the vertebral bodies to approximate. Release of the external pressure allows the internal nucleus pressure to again separate the vertebral end-plates and restore the vertebral column length and physiological curves (Fig. 11). Flexion or extension forces deform the nuclei, but release restores the erect curves. The deformation of the nucleus is compression with maintenance of its cubic content. The annulus "bulges" peripherally.

Attrition of aging and repeated stresses cause dehydration of both nucleus and annulus with fragmentation of annulus circumferential fibers (Fig. 12). The vertebrae approximate and the longitudinal ligaments become slack. Asymmetrical degeneration of the intervertebral disks can occur, resulting in abnormal alignment of the vertebral column. The significance of disk degeneration upon adult scoliosis will be discussed in Chapter 7.

In the posterior aspect of the functional units of the vertebral column are found the posterior joints—the facets. The facets are curved, cartilage-covered joints that bear little or no weight when the spine is erect. They are in close proximity to the

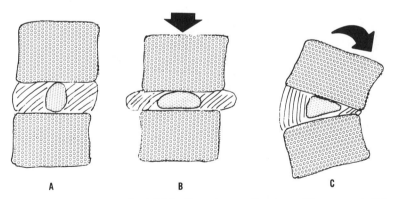

A   B   C

FIGURE 11. Intervertebral Disk: Reaction to Pressure. The normal disk with rounded intact nucleus (A) maintains vertebral separation. Compression deforms the nucleus and "bulges" the annulus physiologically (B). Flexion or extension deforms the disk nucleus and permits the motion (C). Upon release of compression or bending forces, the disk resumes its normal position as a result of the intrinsic intervertebral disk pressure.

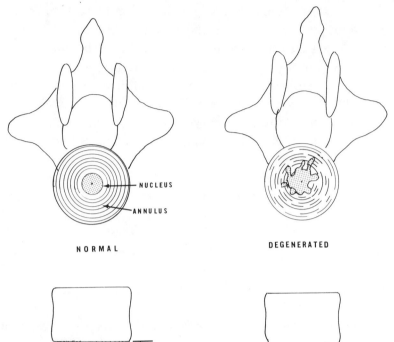

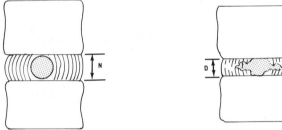

NORMAL

DEGENERATED

NUCLEUS

ANNULUS

FIGURE 12. Intervertebral Disk: Degeneration. The normal disk has a well-hydrated nucleus and intact annular fibers with normal interdiskal pressure that maintains normal separation of the vertebral bodies(N). Degeneration of the disk implies dehydration and fragmentation of annular fibers with some radial tearing. The nucleus escapes into adjacent annular fibers and loses its interdiskal pressure, thus allowing the vertebral bodies to approximate (D).

superior facets of the lower vertebral body, opposed to the inferior facets of the more cephalad body, and upon motion, they glide upon each other. By their plane alignment, as has been stated, they direct the direction of motion and simultaneously deny contrary motion.

Scoliosis is unphysiological curving laterally from the midline. Owing to vertebral alignment and the structural relationships of the vertebral borders and the posterior articulation,

16

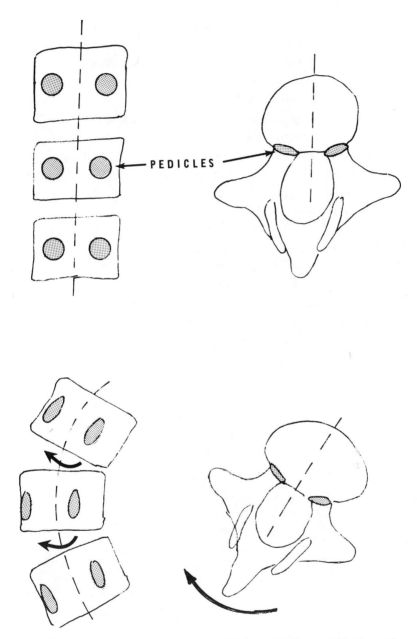

PEDICLES

FIGURE 13. Simultaneous Rotation of Spine with Lateral Flexion. The erect spine without scoliosis has no vertebral rotation. The symmetry of the pedicles from the midline ascertain this **(top)**. As the spine laterally flexes, the vertebrae rotate toward the convex side **(bottom)**.

lateral bending is accompanied by simultaneous rotation (Fig. 13). The exact engineering principle of this associated rotation is not fully understood, but the rotation occurs with significant stress in the structural scoliosis to gradually cause deformation of the vertebral units (the bodies, the facets, and the posterior arches). Since there is rotation of the thoracic spine associated with lateral curving, the ribs, by virtue of their unyielding attachment to the vertebrae, also undergo stress and structural deformation. Their angulation and form is altered in scoliosis, causing much of the thoracic cosmetic deformity.

A rib articulates with the thoracic vertebrae at two points: the head of the rib articulates with the vertebral body, and the tubercle of the rib articulates with the transverse process. Because of its position it passes the intervertebral disk space. The rib is firmly attached to the vertebral body and the transverse process by the capsular ligaments and is reinforced by the costovertebral ligament and the costotransversal ligament (Fig. 14). These ligaments came under intensive study when

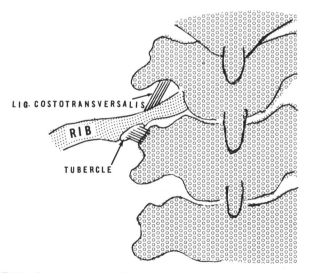

FIGURE 14. Costovertebral Ligaments. Ligaments connect the tubercle of the rib to the vertebral body. A short, strong costotransversalis ligament binds the rib to the adjacent transverse process of the more cephalad vertebra.

18

they were thought to be instrumental in the causation of scoliosis and the advocated treatment was to resect them. This therapy has been largely refuted.

Scoliosis is by definition lateral rotatory deforming curving of the spine. It is one of the major spinal diseases in growing children. Many terms are involved in defining scoliosis and many types are recognized. The Scoliosis Research Society, an affiliate of the American Academy of Orthopaedic Surgeons, has standardized a glossary of scoliosis terms which hopefully will have universal acceptance and utilization so that international statistics will be meaningful. Chapter 3 is devoted to this glossary and contains a brief practical explanation of most terms.

CHAPTER 3

Glossary of Scoliosis Terms

Many terms have been used in medical terminology with inconsistent understanding and nouniformity. The glossary, formulated by the Scoliosis Research Society, will have international utilization once it is accepted. Such a universally accepted glossary has been needed to ensure uniform understanding of diagnosis and of treatment results.

SITE OF CURVES

Scoliosis is specified by its anatomical site in the vertebral column. The spine is normally divided into the cervical, thoracic, and lumbar spines (Fig. 15). Viewed laterally, the physiological curves are lordosis of the cervical and lumbar with kyphosis at the thoracic and sacral segments. The terminology of "scoliosis curves," however, implies a curve viewed anteriorly-posteriorly and must be considered pathological.

A *cervical* curve has its apex from C_1 to C_6, a *thoracic* curve its apex between T_2 and T_{12} with a *cervicothoracic* curve arbitrarily having its apex at C_7 or T_1. A *lumbar* curve has its apex between L_1 and L_4; a curve that has its apex at T_{12} or L_1 is considered a *thoracolumbar* curve. A curve with its apex at L_5 or below is termed a *lumbosacral* curve. The significance of

21

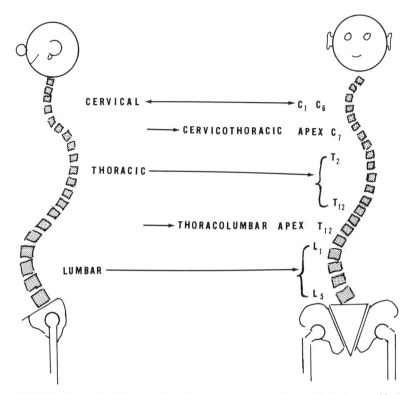

FIGURE 15. Spinal Level of Scoliosis Curvatures. The scoliosis is specified to exist at the spinal level related to either the cervical, cervicothoracic, thoracic, thoracolumbar, or lumbar vertebrae (or to more than one of such levels). These levels are depicted in this illustration.

specifying the vertebral area of the scoliosis curve is that each site and extent of scoliosis curvature has a therapeutic and prognostic significance. The site of curvature along with the associated history, age, and sex of the patient contributes to its diagnostic and prognostic status.

Since there are also laterally viewed curvatures of a pathological significance when they exceed physiological degrees or are associated with the preceding scoliotic curve, they are now standardized into two types.

(A) *Kyphos* is an increase in the posterior convex angulation of the spine in the sagittal plane. Twenty to forty degrees of kyphosis is considered a normal range (Fig. 16). When exces-

22

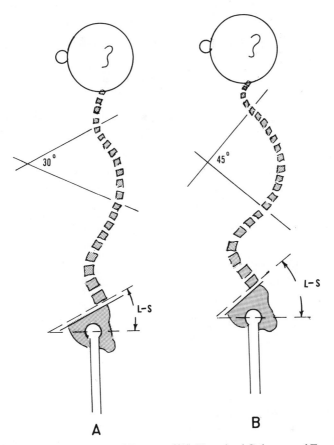

FIGURE 16. Normal Lateral Curves of the Vertebral Column and Excessive
Kyphosis and Lordosis. A shows the normal spine, which has a dorsal
kyphosis of approximately 30° and minimal lumbar lordosis. Excessive dorsal kyphosis (45° or above) is termed *round back*; when it is combined with
scoliosis (lateral curving), it is called *kyphoscoliosis* (**B**). A kyphos of less
than 20° is also considered abnormal and is termed *dorsal lordoscoliosis*.
Excessive lumbar lordosis has no standardized numerical degree of abnormality, but is only a clinical impression.

sive kyphosis is associated with lateral curvature, it is termed
kyphoscoliosis. A kyphos less than 20° in the thoracic spine
is also considered abnormal and is termed *lordoscoliosis*.

(B) *Lordosis* is a curve with convexity anteriorly and is
physiological. It is considered pathological when excessive,
but no standard numerical degrees are yet designated as

23

pathological. If it is associated with simultaneous scoliosis it is termed *lordoscoliosis*. An increase in anterior curvature is more aptly termed *lordoscoliosis*.

TYPES OF CURVES

Spinal curvatures must be differentiated as *structural* or *functional* (nonstructural). In a structural curve a segment of the spine has a fixed curve that does not correct upon lateral bending or in the supine position. Functional curves may be transient or fairly persistent, but have no structural changes (Fig. 17). These curves correct or overcorrect, and this can be observed in x-rays of patients in a side-bending or prone position.

In viewing a scoliosis curve the *primary* curve can be considered to be the first of several curves to appear. It may be difficult to determine or identify on later studies, and the primary curve may not be the major curve. The *major* curve is

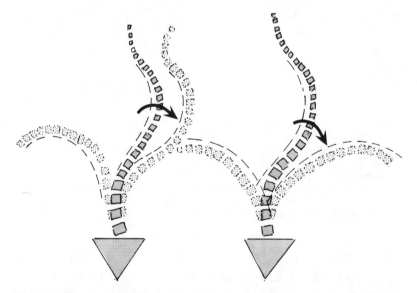

FIGURE 17. Scoliosis Flexibility. The spine in the **left** figure is *in*flexible in that lateral bending does *not* alter or correct the thoracic curvature. This implies a "fixed" scoliosis. The figure to the **right** depicts curvature correction upon lateral bending implying functional flexibility and absence of structural changes.

24

the largest curve with the greatest angulation. The growing spine usually attempts to maintain balance with body alignment (Fig. 18).

A *secondary* or *compensatory* curve usually develops above or below the major curve in an attempt to maintain normal body alignment. The aim of treatment, either conservative or surgical, in addition to decreasing the degree of curve, is to achieve and/or regain and to maintain alignment.

Balanced or compensatory curves align the midpoint of the occiput directly over the sacrum: This alignment is determined

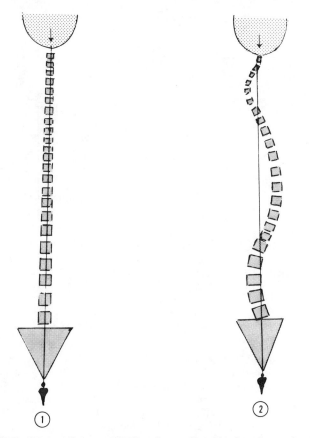

FIGURE 18. Body Alignment. Normally an aligned spine shows the occiput aligned directly over the sacrum as measured by a plumb line (**1**). In scoliosis, in spite of curvature, the relationship of occiput to pelvis should be one of balanced alignment (**2**).

25

clinically by a plumb line. Roentgenologically the sum of the angular deviations of the spine in one direction are equal to those in the opposite direction (thoracic=lumbar) (Fig. 19).

The *minor curve* is a term used to refer to the smaller of the

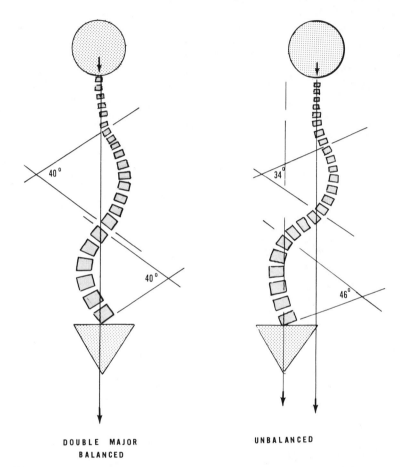

DOUBLE MAJOR
BALANCED

UNBALANCED

FIGURE 19. Double Major Curves: Major Double Minor Curves. A double major curve is a scoliosis where both curves are of equal degree of angulation and each balances the other. A major curve may be balanced by two minor curves. The minor curves may be double or single and are considered *compensatory* curves. The scoliosis of the figure to the **left** is "balanced" in that the occiput is directly above the pelvis and spine is "plumb level." In the figure to the **right** the scoliosis is unbalanced so that the plumb line from the base of the occiput to the sacrum falls several centimeters to the right of midline. This is a very important clinical test in that "unbalanced" or uncompensated curves tend to progress more and are more difficult to treat.

26

several curves. When there are two structural curves of equal importance the condition is called *double major scoliosis*. The curves in this type of scoliosis are most frequently a thoracic and a somewhat larger lumbar curve (Fig. 19). When both structural curves occur in the thoracic spine, the larger usually

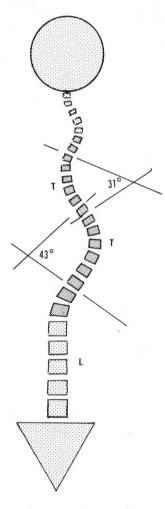

DOUBLE THORACIC

FIGURE 20. Double Thoracic Curves. When both structural curves occur in the thoracic spine, the scoliosis is termed *double thoracic curves*. Usually the major curve is in the lower thoracic spine and the minor or compensatory in the upper thoracic area.

27

occurs in the lower thoracic spine and the lesser in the upper thoracic area (Fig. 20). The lower thoracic curve is usually the more deforming and both thoracic curves may be accompanied by a compensatory nonstructural lumbar curve.

Scoliosis is also differentiated according to the patient's age at onset because of diagnostic and prognostic factors. A spinal curvature developing during the first 3 years of life is termed *infantile;* a curvature developing between the fourth and twelfth year in girls and between the fourth and fourteenth year in boys is termed *juvenile.* A curve developing after the bone age of 12 in girls and 14 in boys, but before maturity, is called *adolescent* scoliosis. The spinal curvature that exists after skeletal maturity is considered *adult* scoliosis.

MEASUREMENT OF CURVES

Curves are currently universally measured by the Cobb method (Fig. 21), as standardized by the Scoliosis Research Society. Previously, curvatures were computed by the Ferguson method, which was considered standard, as well as by the Cobb method. Since there are still Ferguson measurements recorded on many clinic charts, it is necessary to understand them (Fig. 22).

The term *apical vertebra* occurs frequently in scoliosis literature and refers to the most rotated vertebra in a curve. Since most scoliotic curves have some vertebral rotation, measurement of this rotation would be very desirable. There is currently no method of measurement that is universally accepted (Fig. 23). This rotation (Fig. 24) creates the greatest cosmetic defect and, in the thoracic area, cardiopulmonary involvement results as the greatest potential functional impairment.

Rotation occurs posteriorly (the scapular area) on the convex side of the scoliosis and anteriorly on the concave side. This rotational deformity is formed by the rib cage in the thoracic area and by the erector spinae muscles in the lumbar area. In moderate to severe scoliotic curves the rotation is

28

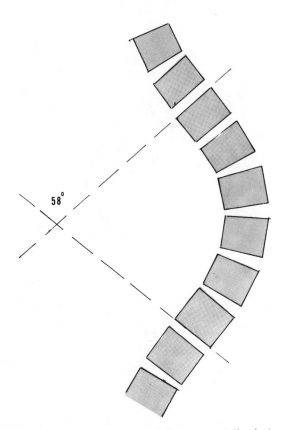

FIGURE 21. Cobb Method of Measuring Curvature. A line is drawn perpendicular to the upper margin of the vertebra which inclines most toward the concavity. A line is also drawn on the inferior border of the lower vertebra with greatest angulation toward the concavity. The angle of these transecting lines is noted and recorded. The apical vertebra is noted but does not enter into the measurement.

noted by protrusion of the posterior rib cage and the overlying scapula (humping or "razor back"). In smaller and in early curves the rotation can only be noted when the patient is observed while he is bent forward at the hip to a 90° angle (Figs. 25 and 26).

Since examining the patient in this position reveals early minimal curves, this is the recommended method of routine examination for all children so that scoliosis may be discovered in its early stages. This method of examination is recom-

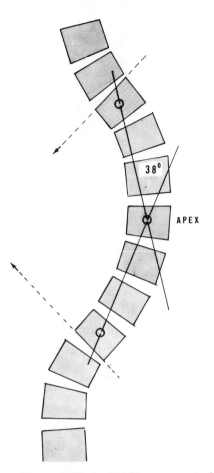

FIGURE 22. Risser-Ferguson Method of Measurement of Scoliosis Curve.
To measure the degrees of scoliosis curvature the method of Risser-Ferguson
is still occasionally used but no longer is internationally accepted. The diskal
vertebra is the lowest vertebra whose inferior surface tilts to the concavity of
the curve; the proximal vertebra is the highest one whose superior surface
tilts to the cavity of the curve. Lines transect the middle of the apical
vertebra, and the angle is measured from these transecting lines.

mended to parents, teachers, nurses, physical educators, etc.,
as well as to physicians. Curvatures that indicate existing
structural changes will thus be discovered by examination of
the spine of the flexed patient before they are observable in the
erect patient.

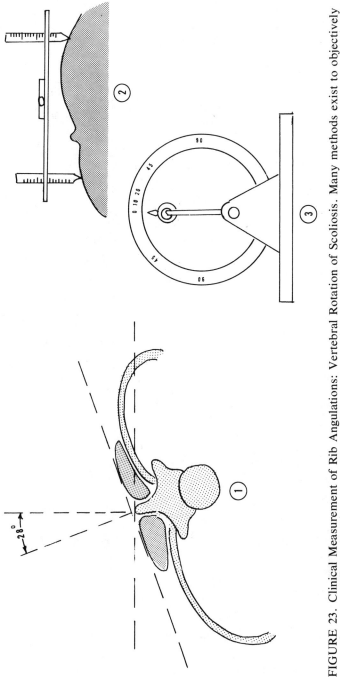

FIGURE 23. Clinical Measurement of Rib Angulations: Vertebral Rotation of Scoliosis. Many methods exist to objectively measure rotational deformity of the scoliotic spine. 1 depicts the rib angulation related to thoracic vertebral rotation. 2 is an instrument that can be read from the scales on the convex and the concave side of the rib cage that when compared to horizontal gives a numerical reading. In the scale depicted in 3 the swinging needle is buoyed by an air bubble, and the angle of obliquity is read directly on the circular scale in degrees from true vertical 0°.

31

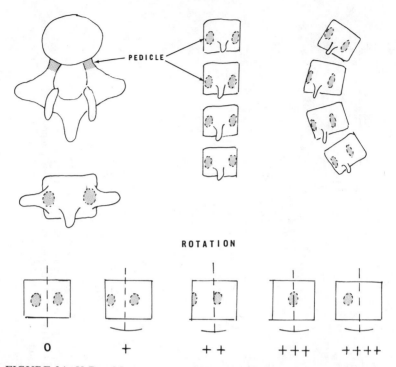

ROTATION

0	+	+ +	+ + +	+ + + +

FIGURE 24. X-Ray Measurement of Vertebral Rotation. By observing the pedicles on the spine x-ray (**top**), it can be seen that their relationship to the midline forms a scale of 0 to 4 (**bottom**). This scale is not yet universally standardized and is only used in some clinics. Once used, however, it affords comparison for subsequent examinations.

VERTEBRAL BODY CHANGES

Insofar as scoliosis is prevalent and most progressive among "growing" children, the implication is that vertebral bodies not yet completed in growth allow for the progression of scoliosis. Thus an understanding of the growth pattern of vertebral bodies is necessary.

The vertebral bodies are composed of the diaphysis and the vertebral *end-plates*, which are the superior and inferior plates of cortical bone of the body adjacent to the disk space (Fig. 27). The vertebral *growth plates* are the cartilaginous surfaces circling the top and bottom of the body and are composed of

32

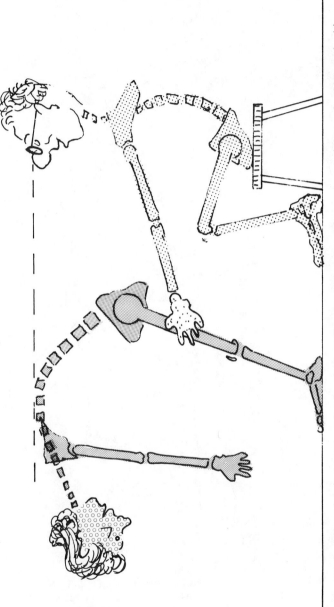
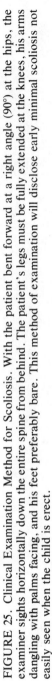

FIGURE 25. Clinical Examination Method for Scoliosis. With the patient bent forward at a right angle (90°) at the hips, the examiner sights horizontally down the entire spine from behind. The patient's legs must be fully extended at the knees, his arms dangling with palms facing, and his feet preferably bare. This method of examination will disclose early minimal scoliosis not easily seen when the child is erect.

33

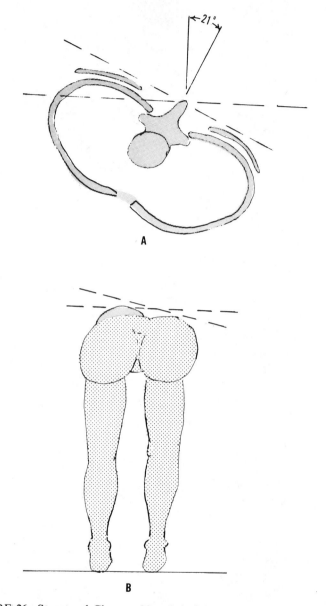

FIGURE 26. Structural Changes Noted during Examination. Viewing the bent-over patient from a posterior aspect (Fig. 25) will reveal rotational changes in rib angulation (**A**) not always noted in erect posture. The rib angulation is noted clinically as a "rib hump" on the convex side (**B**).

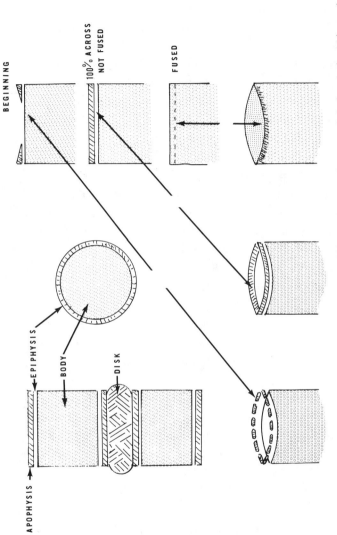

FIGURE 27. Vertebral Apophyseal Growth. The figure to the left depicts the apophyses and their relationship to the vertebral bodies. They are separated by the epiphyseal growth centers. Growth begins with fragments of apophysis that eventually merge into a complete ring and ultimately fuse with the vertebral body. At the stage of fusion, further vertebral growth ceases. Clinically the growth potential is graded as "beginning," "across but not fused," to completely fused. The degree of union of the apophyseal segments (stated as a percentage) is 100%.

35

apophysis and epiphysis. The unfused growth plates are visible in routine x-rays, but with some difficulty in anterior-posterior views. They are best seen on oblique views. The iliac apophyses were determined to parallel vertebral end-plate growth. Since these are readily visible and measurable they are used to determine the remaining growth potential of the spine. Measurement of the iliac apophysis is by the so-called Risser sign. In an anterior-posterior x-ray of the pelvis, when the iliac apophysis beginning at the anterior-superior spine crosses over the crest and reaches the junction of the ilia and the sacrum and the epiphysis closes, vertebral growth is considered to be complete, and no further vertebral growth is expected (Fig. 28).

Of academic interest but of no significance regarding completion of vertebral growth is the determination of *skeletal bone age*. This age is determined by comparing anterior-posterior x-rays of the left hand and wrist with the standards of the Greulich and Pyle atlas.[1] Of equal insignificance with regard to cessation of vertebral growth is the age of onset of menses. There is no documented correlation of the cessation of vertebral growth with the skeletal bone age or the onset of menses.

LEG LENGTH

Since the spine is vertically dependent upon the horizontality of the pelvis, an oblique sacral base can produce a superincumbent scoliosis. Pelvic obliquity can be due to contracture either above or below the pelvis or due to inequality of leg length. The superincumbent scoliosis attributable to a pelvic obliquity is usually functional (Fig. 29). There is no evidence that this functional scoliosis becomes structural with passage of time in an uncorrected leg-length discrepancy.

Leg length may be unequal because of asymmetrical growth of otherwise normal femur or tibia, hip pathology, moderate or severe varus or valgus, or post-traumatic residual deformity.

Clinical evaluation can usually elicit the pelvic obliquity. By

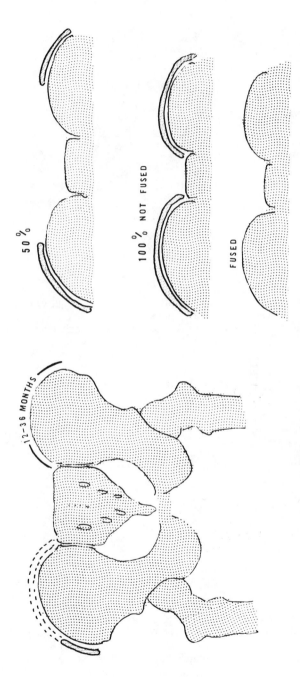

FIGURE 28. Iliac Apophyseal Evaluation of Remaining Vertebral Growth. The vertebral body epiphyseal centers are not always discernable or measurable on routine anterior-posterior views. Risser estimated that growth of the iliac apophyses was equal to vertebral body apophyseal growth and thus, being readily visible, could be used to determine remaining growth. The onset of iliac apophysis begins at the anterior superior spine of the ilium and proceeds medially to the sacroiliac joint. A time factor of 12 to 36 months is expected for complete excursion. So long as there is further excursion and no fusion noted, further spine growth can be expected and thus more progression of the scoliosis is possible. So long as there is further growth potention, treatment as well as periodic observation must continue.

37

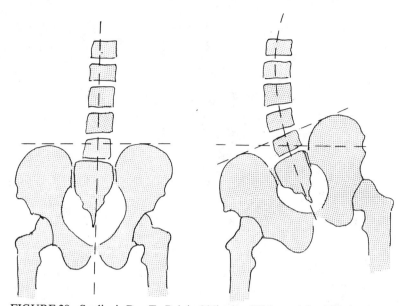

FIGURE 29. Scoliosis Due To Pelvic Obliquity. With a pelvic obliquity due to a unilateral short leg, regardless of cause, the spine can assume a scoliosis **(right)**. This is created by the attempt of the spine to assume balance to the center of gravity.

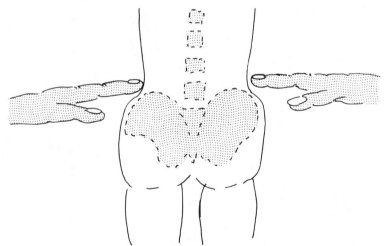

FIGURE 30. Clinical Evaluation of Pelvic Level. With the examiner's hands placed on the brim of the patient's pelvic crests, the patient, while standing erect, is viewed from behind. The level of the iliac crests can thus be determined. An obliquity can be ascertained and its degree determined by placing a board of known thickness under the "short" leg and reexamining the crest level.

38

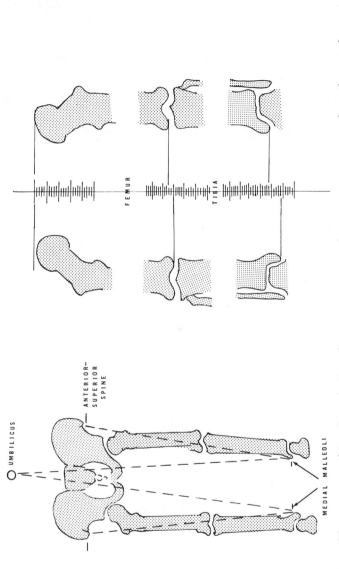

FIGURE 31. Exact Measurement of Leg Length. By using a tape measure the exact measurement from the anterior-superior spine to the medial ankle malleoli can be measured. Confirmation is possible by measuring from the umbilicus to the malleoli. Exact x-ray measurement can be made by a scanogram (depicted on the **right**) where exact differences can be measured in millimeters on the scale of the x-ray plate.

39

observing the standing patient from a rear view, the iliac crest can be ascertained and a gross discrepancy noted (Fig. 30). Leg-length discrepancy can be measured accurately by observing a board of known thickness under the foot of the suspected short leg and then determining the pelvic level. Exact measurements of leg length can be obtained by scanogram (Fig. 31) or clinically by tape measure. A discrepancy of less than ¾ inch rarely needs correction by orthopaedic shoe lift and does not adversely affect the scoliosis.

Reference

1. W. W. Greulich, and S. I. Pyle: Radiographic Atlas of the Hand and Wrist, ed. 2. Stanford University Press, California, 1959.

CHAPTER 4

Types of Scoliosis and Theories of Etiology

TYPES OF SCOLIOSIS

The classification of spine deformity is being standardized by the Committee of Classification of the Scoliosis Research Society. As new types and new variants are found they are listed in the classification. It is apparent from this list that scoliosis accompanies many diseases and abnormalities.

Classification of Spine Deformity

I. Idiopathic
   A. Infantile (very rare in the U.S.A.)
      1. Resolving: This type of curve has the ability to resolve, but this rarely occurs in deformities of later onset.
      2. Progressive
   B. Juvenile
   C. Adolescent
II. Neuromuscular
   A. Neuropathic (neurogenic); due to disease or anomalies of nerve tissue
      1. Upper motor neuron lesion
         a. Cerebral palsy

        b. Spinocerebellar degeneration disease
           (1) Friedreich's
           (2) Charcot-Marie-Tooth
           (3) Roussy-Lévy
        c. Syringomyelia
        d. Spinal cord tumor
        e. Spinal cord trauma
        f. Other
    2. Lower motor neuron lesion
        a. Poliomyelitis
        b. Other viral myelitis
        c. Traumatic
        d. Spinal muscular atrophy disease
           (1) Werdnig-Hoffmann
           (2) Kugelberg-Welander
        e. Myelomeningocoele (paralytic)
    3. Dysautonomia (Riley-Day syndrome)
    4. Other
  B. Myopathic (myogenic); due to disease or anomalities of the musculature
    1. Arthrogryposis
    2. Muscular dystrophy
        a. Duchenne's (pseudohypertrophic)
        b. Limb-girdle
        c. Facioscapulohumeral
    3. Fiber type disproportion
    4. Congenital hypotonia
    5. Myotonia dystrophica
    6. Other
III. Congenital (due to congenital anomalies of vertebrae or developmental abnormality of the vertebral elements and/or adjacent ribs, acquired or congenital)
  A. Congenital Scoliosis
    1. Failure of formation
        a. Wedge vertebrae
        b. Hemivertebrae

2. Failure of segmentation
   a. Unilateral bar
   b. Bilateral bar ("fusion")
3. Mixed
B. Congenital Kyphosis
   1. Failure of formation
   2. Failure of segmentation
   3. Mixed
C. Congenital Lordosis
D. Associated with Neural Tissue Defect
   1. Myelomeningocoele
   2. Meningocoele
   3. Spinal dysraphism
      a. Diastematomyelia
      b. Other

IV. Neurofibromatosis (suggested by the presence of cafe au lait spots—light brown irregular areas of skin pigmentation).

V. Mesenchymal
   A. Marfan's syndrome
   B. Homocystinuria
   C. Ehlers-Danlos syndrome
   D. Other

VI. Traumatic
   A. Fracture or dislocation (non-paralytic)
   B. Post-irradiation
   C. Post-laminectomy
   D. Other

VII. Soft-Tissue Contractures
   A. Post-empyema
   B. Burn
   C. Other

VIII. Osteochondrodystrophies
   A. Achondroplasia
   B. Spondyloepiphyseal dysplasia

        C. Disastrophic dwarfism
        D. Mucopolysaccharidosis
   IX. Scheuermann's Disease
    X. Infection
        A. Tuberculosis
        B. Bacterial
        C. Fungal
        D. Parasitic
        E. Other
   XI. Tumor
        A. Benign
        B. Malignant
  XII. Rheumatoid Disease
        A. Juvenile
        B. Adult
        C. Strümpell-Marie
 XIII. Metabolic
        A. Ricketts
        B. Juvenile osteoporosis
        C. Osteogenesis imperfecta
  XIV. Related to Lumbosacral Area
        A. Spondylolisthesis
        B. Spondylolysis
        C. Other congenital anomaly
        D. Other
   XV. Thoracogenic (attributable to disease or operative
        trauma in or on the thoracic cage)
        A. Post-empyema
        B. Post-thoracoplasty
        C. Post-thoracotomy
        D. Other
  XVI. Hysterical
 XVII. Functional
        A. Postural
        B. Secondary to short leg
        C. Other

THEORIES OF ETIOLOGY

Although intensive research is being carried out throughout the world the etiology and pathogenics of scoliosis remain unknown. Eighty percent of scoliosis is classified as idiopathic. Statistically, an estimated 4 adolescent girls in 1000 have scoliosis, and approximately 1 in 2,500 boys has scoliosis of some type. Approximately 2 percent of the adult population is estimated to have a certain degree of scoliosis with 0.5 percent having more than a 20° curve.

Scoliosis is considered to be potentially progressive during the vertebral growth years, which are those up to age 15 in girls and up to approximately 17 in boys. Which type of scoliosis and what factors are of prognostic significance in determining which patient will progress remains obscure. This unpredictable prognosis makes careful observation at periodic periods of growth mandatory so that any significant increase in curvature can be readily noted and treated. One observation is not usually informative. Idiopathic scoliosis which constitutes approximately 80 percent of all scoliosis is now considered a familial type of curvature. Congenital malformations causing scoliosis are more pathognomonically understandable. Most other types are unexplainable.

Farkas in 1954[1] postulated a pathological separation of the epiphyseal vertebral ring to be pathognomonic, but most authors consider these vertebral changes to be secondary and related to the Hueter-Volkmann principle. However, the internal forces causing enactment of this principle remain unknown. Increased pressure on a vertebral epiphyseal growth plate retards its rate of growth. The unpressured portion grows normally or comparatively more. This growth influences the endochondral ossification and results in "wedging" of the vertebra. (See Fig. 32)

X-ray irradiation (such as that used in the treatment of Willias renal tumor) can cause asymmetric epiphseal growth. Injury to the epiphysis can alter growth and result in secondary

45

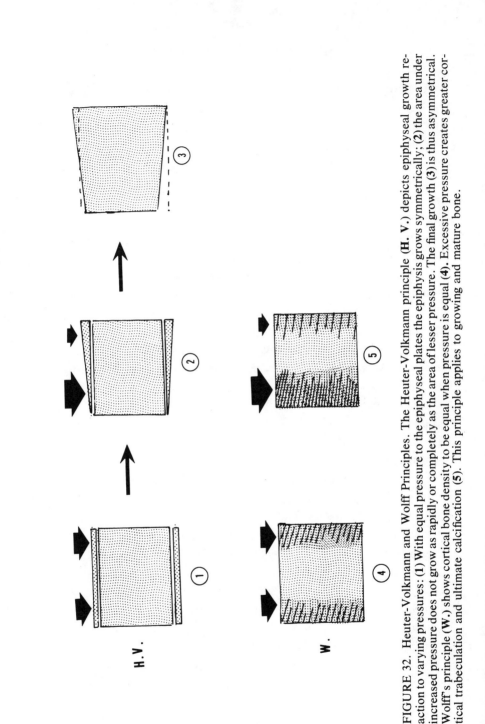

FIGURE 32. Heuter-Volkmann and Wolff Principles. The Heuter-Volkmann principle (**H. V.**) depicts epiphyseal growth reaction to varying pressures: (**1**) With equal pressure to the epiphyseal plates the epiphysis grows symmetrically; (**2**) the area under increased pressure does not grow as rapidly or completely as the area of lesser pressure. The final growth (**3**) is thus asymmetrical. Wolff's principle (**W.**) shows cortical bone density to be equal when pressure is equal (**4**). Excessive pressure creates greater cortical trabeculation and ultimate calcification (**5**). This principle applies to growing and mature bone.

scoliosis, but vertebral fractures are not considered to be a frequent cause of scoliosis. Musculature imbalance as is noted in asymmetrical poliomyelitis paresis has long been known to cause scoliosis. Other causes of muscle imbalance have been investigated to determine their possible influence on the causation of scoliosis. Electromyographic studies on paraspinous muscles in idiopathic scoliosis have failed to reveal any significant changes on the muscles on either the convex or concave side of the curvature. Rotator muscle imbalance has been implicated but never confirmed as a causative factor. Nervous system control of balance was incriminated by Yamada and others[2] in 1969; they believed scoliosis to be more frequent and more severe in children with proprioceptive postural disturbances. Further studies are being conducted in this area. In 1968 MacEwen[3] caused scoliosis in animals by dividing the posterior sensory nerve root but his experiments have subsequently been questioned.

Ligamentous abnormality that causes asymmetrical growth has been incriminated. Experimental section of the costovertebral ligaments has caused scoliosis in quadripeds and when performed on the contralateral side of the spine benefited the scoliosis by decreasing the angulation. This procedure remains equivocal in regard to its benefit and currently is not advocated for use in humans. There is increasing evidence of hereditary factors in scoliosis that indicates idiopathic scoliosis is an inherited disease with possible sex linkage. This evidence appears so probable that the Scoliosis Research Society is considering substituting the term *familial* for the term *idiopathic*.

A cause of scoliosis is attributed to spinal reaction to stressful forces such as gravity or ligamentous muscular action, as explained in Wolff's principle. Wolff's principle as restated by Jansen in 1920 is: "The form of a bone being given, the bone elements place or displace themselves in the direction of functional forces and increase or decrease their mass to reflect the amount of the functional forces."[4] This applies not only to bone, but also to all connective tissues containing collagen and polysaccharide cells. Osteoblasts must be sensitive to variations in pressure and tension. Just how Wolff's principle applies to forces and what its relationship is to scoliosis is not known. Many studies of metabolic and chemical factors have revealed defects related to scoliosis that have interesting possibilities, but to date none have been corraborated. It has been speculated, in this regard, that scoliosis is a form of unborn error of metabolism where the only clinical sign is a curvature of the spine, but until this metabolic effect is found it does not yield a diagnostic or therapeutic rationale. Since currently no consistent, confirmed cause is known for idiopathic scoliosis and not all the mechanisms of the better-known causes are understood, diagnosis of scoliosis remains a clinical one, and treatment remains aimed at prevention or correction of existing curvatures.

References

1. A. Farkas: The pathogenesis of idiopathic scoliosis. J. Bone Joint Surg. [Am.] 36:617, 1954.
2. K. Yamada et al.: Equilibrium function in scoliosis and active corrective plaster jacket for the treatment. Tokushima J. Exp. Med. 16:1, 1969.
3. G. D. MacEwen: Experimental scoliosis. *In* Proceedings of a Second Symposium on Scoliosis: Causation, P. A. Zorab (Ed.), Longman Group LTD, London, 1969, p. 18.
4. T. Zuk: The etiology and pathogenesis of idiopathic scoliosis from the viewpoint of the electromyographic studies (abs.). Beitr. Orthop. Traumatol. 12:138, 1965.

CHAPTER 5

Recognition and Diagnosis

In many instances potential scoliosis will first be diagnosed incidentally or even accidentally. Because symptoms in early scoliosis are minimal or even absent, it is understandable that discovery may not be made until deforming scoliosis is already present. *This fact is the basis of massive international education programs being initiated to ensure early recognition of scoliosis before irreversible changes occur.*

SYMPTOMS

If no symptoms occur in early scoliosis, the question can be raised, "Why the urgency of early diagnosis for early treatment?" There are three significant residual effects of scoliosis that justify treatment: (1) cosmesis; (2) pain; and (3) cardiopulmonary symptoms.

Abnormal appearance due to the presence of scoliosis is the usual reason for the seeking of medical evaluation by a child's parents. Ultimately the unsightly appearance from the deformity caused by scoliosis is of greatest concern to the patient. Pain attributable to scoliosis is not prevalent or initially severe and occurs mostly in the low back when lumbar scoliosis is marked. Associated dorsal kyphosis can cause upper back pain as excessive lumbar lordosis can cause low back pain, but again, pain is rare. Undesirable postural appearance is the most common symptom of excessive dorsal kyphosis. Cardiorespiratory symptoms are rarely seen in scoliosis of less than 50°, and they are especially more likely to occur when the scoliosis is in the thoracic or thoracolumbar regions.

Since cosmesis is the predominant symptom, early or moderate spinal curvature is often first noted by a parent or relative. It may be discovered by a school nurse or physical education instructor in a routine school examination or during summer months when the child is more likely to be unclothed at such places as beaches or swimming pools. It may first be noticed during an annual pediatric examination by an alert pediatrician or family practitioner. Not infrequently it is noted on an x-ray taken to aid other diagnoses and may be discovered through a routine chest x-ray, abdominal x-rays, or x-ray films taken following trauma.

"Poor posture," "one shoulder higher," or "one shoulder blade protruding" can bring the patient under direct observation. Ill-fitting clothing due to scoliosis is a possible initial complaint, but at the usual age of onset of scoliosis this would be unlikely.

Since poor posture or some other possible evidence of scoliosis is not noted by the child and frequently is not seen by parents who rarely see their child undressed or standing still, the condition often becomes progressive before it is discovered.

The symptom of thoracic or lumbar pain is so infrequent, especially in early and mild scoliosis, that this symptom warrants search for other causative factors. Unless scoliosis is very severe and of long duration, shortness of breath, orthopnea, and excessive fatigue also demand thorough evaluation for other causes.

EXAMINATION

To uncover and evaluate scoliosis it is necessary that the child be examined in the upright posture and in sufficient degree of undress. Both feet must be parallel and both knees fully extended. To examine a child standing with one knee slightly bent can cause a pelvic obliquity and a superincumbent "functional" scoliosis. All postural aspects of the child during the examination must be supervised and correct so that the examination is meaningful.

The level of the pelvis can be determined by direct vision by placing the examiner's finger tips on the iliac crest and viewing the pelvic horizontality at arm's length, as was seen in Figure 30. A difference of as slight as ¼ inch can be ascertained by this examination.

The "balance" of the spine can be easily detected by a surveyor's plumb line. The string is held at the base of the occiput and the plumb weight below the gluteal crease; the lower end of the string bisects the sacrum. The lateral deviation of the string from the midline can be accurately measured and should be recorded. The measurement can be recorded on a special scoliosis record and also noted on the x-ray. Since treatment is aimed at resuming or maintaining exact plumb-level balance, these measurements are meaningful. (See Figs. 18 and 19.) Not infrequently scoliosis does not appear in the erect, standing child, but upon examination with the spine flexed forward, an incipient scoliosis becomes apparent. Forward flexion of the thoracic spine accentuates or reveals a thoracic scoliosis often not recognized in the standing erect position. This fact demands *that all children whose spine is examined must be viewed from behind in a 90° forward stance position, both arms dependent ("hanging loosely"), palms facing each other, both legs parallel, and knees fully extended.* (See Fig. 26.) Emphasizing this to any person entrusted with examining children will reveal early mild curvature.

The elbows bent at 90° with the arms dependent at the child's body should be horizontally level with the iliac crests (Fig. 33).

Skin folds at the waist are deeper and more numerous on the concave side of the scoliosis. The posterior superior spine can be palpated and alignment noted both in the standing and

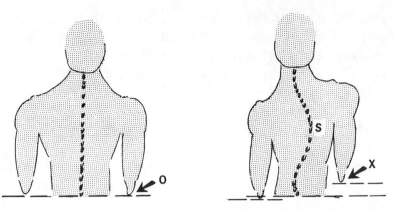

FIGURE 33. Elbow Level in Evaluation of Scoliosis. With the child standing erect and with the arms bent 90° at the elbows, the level of the elbows should be horizontal if the spine is straight (O). Spinal curvature (S) will alter the level of the elbows (X).

bent-over positions. The level of the scoliosis and its apical vertebra can be estimated by clinical evaluation, but can only be confirmed exactly through specific x-ray examination.

MEASUREMENT AND DIAGNOSIS

Upon discovering a scoliosis the exact site can be determined clinically (e.g., thoracic, lumbar), with confirmation again accomplished by x-ray. The flexibility of the curve, which will have prognostic significance, should also be determined. This can be done by lateral bending of the patient and observation by the examiner of reversal of the curves. A functional curve will correct partially or completely upon lateral flexion, whereas no significant correction occurs upon lateral flexion of the structural scoliotic curve. Flexible scoliosis has a better prognosis from adequate treatment than does an inflexible curve.

Since most scoliotic spines have some degree of deforming vertebral rotation, this must be noted, measured, and recorded. This rotatory deformity is more apparent and deforming in the thoracic spine because of the rib deformities that accompany the vertebral rotation. No method of measurement has yet been standardized, but some common method should be instituted by all clinics so that their repeated examinations objectively reveal progression or failure of progression of the rotation. The benefits of treatment relative to rotation can be demonstrated by comparison of previous measurements.

The flexibility of the scoliosis curve, its reversibility, and thus its correctability, can be evaluated by applying traction to the head and neck in the standing position. An assistant can place his hand at the base of the occiput and under the chin and manually "lift" the patient. The observer can evaluate grossly if the curves are fixed or flexible by their change during this traction. No exact measurement of the correction is possible by this method—merely an impression of "flexibility"—and its value is far less than that of lateral-bending examination clinically and on x-rays.

Ultimately accurate diagnosis of type, location, extent, apex, and exact measurement of the curves require accurate x-ray evaluation of the erect spine. Routine x-rays on a 14 × 17 inch film, which is a standard diagnostic film usually taken of the prone patient, does not give full evaluation. Nor are these views standardized, so films from various clinics or various countries cannot be compared. Also, failure to include the pelvis in the x-ray does not reveal the level or obliquity of the sacral base or the remaining growth evaluation of the iliac apophysis. Without an upright view of the patient, the effect of gravity upon the scoliosis is not observable.

It is now standardized internationally that x-rays be taken on a 36-inch film with the anode at a distance of 72 inches. For this film to have proper analytic value, the x-ray equipment must have: (1) a one-to-five grid front with focal distance from 36 to 72 inches, 80 lines per inch; (2) a rotatory anode at a distance of 72 inches; (3) a 0 to 4 aluminum wedge filter to bring about the "heel effect." The patient must stand erect with both feet preferably bare and both knees fully extended and parallel. The x-ray casette must be placed so as to include the head as well as the pelvis of the patient.

X-ray films must be marked to indicate the right and left sides of the patient and when measured, be done as if the patient were being seen from behind as in the clinical examination. By this, the exact site of the major curve, the compensatory curve, and the apical vertebra can be specified. Diagnosis then of "a right major thoracic curve with apex at the eighth thoracic vertebral (T_8) level involving 10 vertebrae in the curve" is meaningful. Rotation as measured can also become a matter of record. The presence of secondary or compensatory curve or curves can also be so noted and the side specified. To merely rely on the heart shadow to indicate the left side of the chest is not always possible if dextrocardia is present.

As has been previously discussed (Chapter 3, p. 28), the Cobb method of measurement should specify the degree of curvature (see Fig. 21). Whichever measurement of rotation is used by the examiner should also be charted. The apical vertebra can be specified. This is the maximally rotated vertebra of the curve. The number of vertebrae in the curve should also be identified and recorded.

To elicit the generalized flexibility of the child as to constitutionally inflexible or extremely hyperflexible is not easily standardized, but Harrington has devised a flexibility test utilizing the finger extensibility and grading to four degrees of flexibility (Fig. 34).

Progression of scoliosis in a child is possible as long as there remains vertebral growth in the spine. When growth is completed, as indicated by the epiphysis being "closed and fused," vertebral body asymmetry leading to structural scoliosis ceases.

Increase in curvature in adult scoliosis is possible but now is due to intervertebral disk changes with further compression of the disk on the concave side of the curve (Fig. 35). Progression of adult scoliosis is claimed to be approximately one degree per year. However, this progression, in the experience of the au-

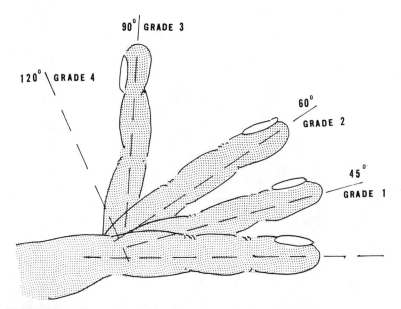

FIGURE 34. Tissue Flexibility: Harrington Criteria. The flexibility of soft tissue is graded from 1 to 4 by hyperextension of the fingers. This is an arbitrary method of determining generalized tissue laxity.

thor, is rare in adult scoliosis except when curves exceed 50°. Some increase is possible in curves of less than 50°, but there is lesser degree of increase and it is much less rapid.

The type of scoliosis and its cause is of diagnostic significance, but, more important, it is of prognostic significance in that it portends the future of the child and can dictate the type and urgency of surgery. Congenital scoliosis with wedge vertebrae or hemivertebrae, for instance, is a candidate for early surgery and must be so considered.

The type of curve or its causative factors may be discovered on the x-ray view. Causes revealed by x-ray may include wedge vertebrae or hemivertebrae (Fig. 36). Failure of segmentation known as congenital bar or, in rare instances, fused vertebrae can also be determined by x-ray view as a cause of scoliosis. The x-rays also determine the extent of remaining bone growth by the degree of epiphyseal closure and fusion. This indicates the expected duration of further growth and thus

55

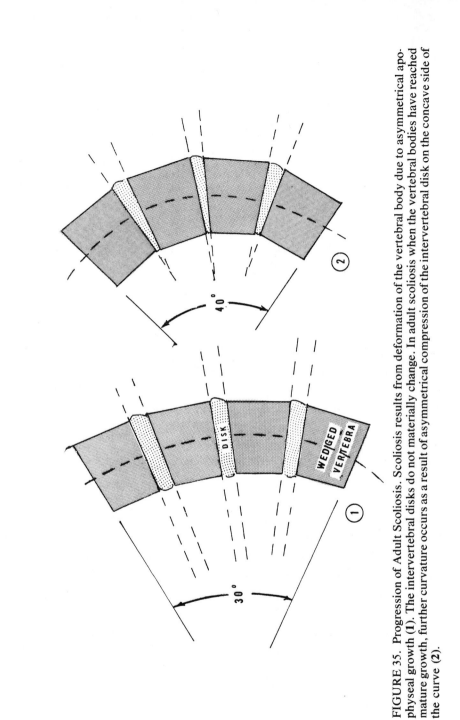

FIGURE 35. Progression of Adult Scoliosis. Scoliosis results from deformation of the vertebral body due to asymmetrical apophyseal growth (1). The intervertebral disks do not materially change. In adult scoliosis when the vertebral bodies have reached mature growth, further curvature occurs as a result of asymmetrical compression of the intervertebral disk on the concave side of the curve (2).

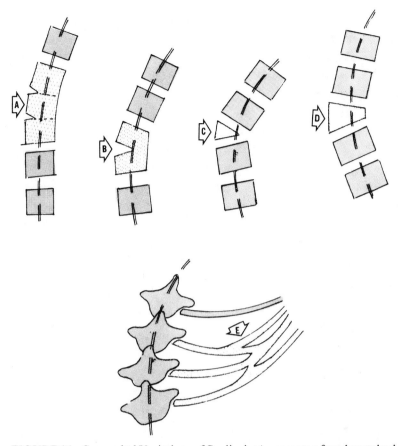

FIGURE 36. Congenital Variations of Scoliosis. **A** presents a fused vertebral segment of three vertebrae; **B** shows segmentation of two vertebrae with a "bar" uniting one half the vertebrae; **C** shows a hemivertebra; and **D** depicts a wedged vertebra. All are congenital causes of scoliosis revealed on x-ray studies. **E** is fusion of ribs that causes a curvature on the concave side of the spine.

the duration of further brace treatment. All treatments, whether by casts or braces, must be continued and supervised during the remaining growth of the child.

Since scoliosis is potentially a progressive condition during bone growth, the iliac crest apophysis, an indicator of bone growth, is significant; its development can be graded in five stages (see Fig. 28).

1. The development of the iliac apophysis has not yet started.
2. The iliac apophysis has started to develop.
3. The iliac apophysis is completely developed.
4. Fusion of the iliac apophysis has started.
5. Fusion to the ileum of the iliac apophysis is completed.

The percentage of each stage of iliac apophyseal growth can be calculated; but the exact remaining period of vertebral growth correlated to the degree of iliac apophysis cannot be ascertained. The original concept that one year of spinal growth remained from the time of appearance of the iliac apophysis (stage 2) until completion of its excursion (stage 3) to the sacroiliac joint is no longer acceptable.

SUMMARY

The most important factor in ensuring early diagnosis of scoliosis is to routinely examine all growing children at regular periods during growth. These periods should preferably be at six-month intervals from early childhood until full maturity with greater attention during the rapid growth phases that usually occur from ages 8 through 12.

Early diagnosis depends on an awareness of its possibility with the hope that early diagnosis will ultimately reveal early minimal scoliosis and result in early referral for treatment. Thus will there be less need for radical surgery to salvage advanced curvature or early surgery, if indicated, will be performed to ensure minimal deformity.

Early scoliosis will be discovered by properly examining the undressed child standing and viewed from behind with the back flexed and the hips bent at 90°. Proper x-rays will establish the degree of curvature, the site and extent of the curve. X-rays will indicate the remaining potential growth and thus the potential progression of the scoliosis. Early discovery of lateral minimal curve before significant rotation has occurred will result in preventing significant cosmetic abnormality, less pain, and preventing cardiopulmonary complication.

A careful history will reveal family incidence, possibly clarify the etiology, and reveal associated congenital conditions.

A worldwide information service is the ultimate hope for uncovering minimal scoliosis while conservative treatment is effective and the prognosis favorable. This service will instruct everyone dealing with children to be alert and, by information service, where and to whom in their vicinity to refer the early scoliotic child for proper care.

CHAPTER 6

Treatment

Over the centuries, many forms of treatment have been advocated for scoliosis, and exponents of every form of treatment are found in the literature. Some aspects and principles of most concepts of treatment have merit and influence today's concept of correct treatment.

The objective of treatment is to ensure that the child reaches maturity with a straight, balanced, and stable spine. In minimal scoliosis that has been diagnosed early, this objective is accomplished by treatment aimed at preventing progression of the deformity. In more advanced cases of scoliosis the treatment objectives are correction of the lateral curving and rotational deformity to the greatest possible degree and holding the correction achieved for the remainder of spinal growth. Treatment either for prevention or correction of scoliosis is either nonoperative or operative. This terminology is preferable to using *conservative* versus *surgical,* since early operative treatment in some forms of scoliosis could be considered conservative. This is exemplified in the early moderate scoliosis that could require four to eight years of bracing or in scoliosis where bracing would merely contain a curve that is moderate but cosmetically unacceptable.

Frequent meaningful examination of a growing child is mandatory. To merely "watch a child progressing in her scoliosis" is inexcusable. It thus behooves any and all individuals whose responsibility it is to examine children to be knowledgeable in the aspects of early discovery of scoliosis. Early referral should be made to a interested physician expert in the treatment of scoliosis. The initial examination of the child to uncover scoliosis falls into the domain of physicians of every specialty who have children under their care. Nurses, physicians' assistants, physical therapists, correction therapists, physical education personnel, and parents share this responsibility.

EXERCISES

The use of exercise has long been advocated in the treatment for scoliosis. Various exercises, including active, passive, symmetrical, asymmetrical, and manipulative exercises, have been expounded. It is currently universally accepted that *exercise alone will not prevent progression of a scoliotic spine, nor will exercise alone correct an existing scoliosis*. Exercises have value in that they may improve posture, increase flexibility, and improve general tone, both muscular and ligamentous. Exercise also has a psychological value in that it improves the feeling of well-being and the self-esteem of the youngster. Exercises performed during the wearing of external devices such as the Milwaukee brace have been proven to be of value, and these will be discussed in this chapter within that context.

EXTERNAL DEVICES

External appliances advocated in the treatment of scoliosis are numerous and many have therapeutic value. These appliances include various forms of traction, plaster casts, braces, and combinations thereof. External devices are either intended to correct curvatures or to maintain correction achieved by other means.

External appliances have their effect on the scoliosis by

application of corrective forces based on the Hueter-Volk-mann and Wolff principles pertaining to the growing spine (see Fig. 32). Generally, pressure is exerted against the convex side of the curve with counterpressure applied against a fixed portion of the skeleton such as the pelvis and rib cage. Pressure is also applied against the convex aspect of rib rotation in an attempt to cause derotation. Traction tends to elongate the spine and thus decrease curvature.

External correction devices can be divided into passive and kinetic in their action. Passive devices apply the principle of steadily applied pressure with no effort required on the part of the patient. Kinetic correction involves active participation by the patient. The passive form of correction is used in the nonoperative-treatment approach but also has significant application in preoperative correction and postoperative maintenance of scoliosis correction. Passive corrective devices include braces and casts.

Passive Correction: Braces and Casts

Braces are constructed of many materials such as leather, metal, or plastic. They may be constructed so as to be worn constantly or they may be removable. Some correction of the scoliosis usually precedes the application of a cast in order that the cast may ensure improvement of the existing curvature or prevention of further progression. Usually, before the achieved correction a cast can be applied and maximum passive correction of the scoliosis attempted (Fig. 37). To do this gravity must be eliminated and the spine elongated. This can be done by placing the patient in the prone or supine position and applying simultaneous pelvic and cervical traction, which will elongate the spine and decrease the curve. This is more successful when the spine is flexible.

Lateral correction is attempted by either localized pressure plates or by traction straps. Traction and lateral corrective forces are best applied by casting the patient on a scoliosis

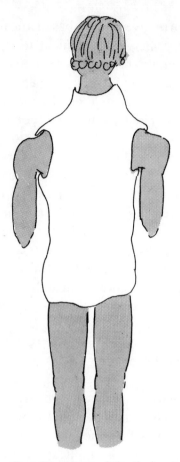

FIGURE 37. Plaster Cast Treatment of Scoliosis. A molded plaster-cast jacket is fitted over a stockinette with the arms exposed. The bottom of the cast molds to the pelvis to control the lordosis. Usually there is a cephalad extension to include the neck and thus effect the thoracic spine. This type of casting is usually applied to hold the correction gotten by other methods such as traction or localizer casts.

frame. There are many designs for these frames, but they all employ the same principles (Fig. 38).

Plaster correction of scoliosis has been used for many years. Plaster casting has had many treatment objectives—from correction of the curves to prevention of further progression after correction by other methods. A favored cast method has employed cutting a wedge in the cast on the convex side of the

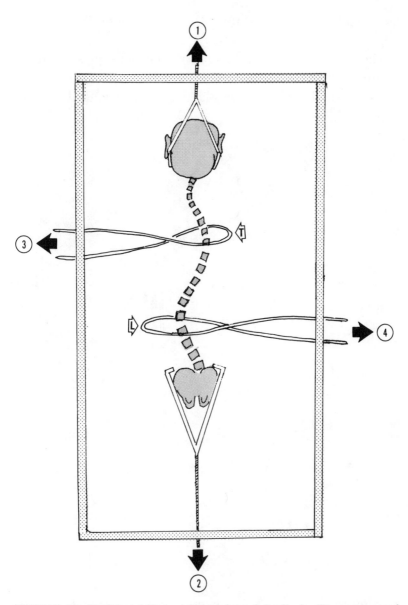

FIGURE 38. Horizontal Frame Correction of Scoliosis. The purpose of frame traction in the treatment of scoliosis is the elimination of gravity and the elongation of the spine. Cervical traction (1) with counter pelvic traction (2) elongates the spine. Lateral straps used as localizer forces pull laterally against the thoracic (3) and lumbar (4) convexity. Rotation may also be included in the corrective forces by placing the lateral straps above or below the horizontal level of the frame.

curve and approximating the segments with a turnbuckle (Fig. 39).

The advantages of passive correction with plaster are its relatively low cost and the fact that skin-tight correction is maximum and is continuously applied. The beneficial effect of

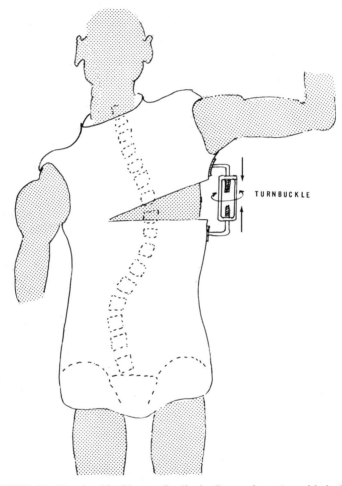

TURNBUCKLE

FIGURE 39. Turnbuckle Plaster Scoliosis Correction. A molded plaster body jacket is applied to the patient while he is reclining on a frame to eliminate gravity; frame traction elongates the spine so that the scoliosis is partially corrected while the cast is being applied. A wedge is cut in the cast on the convex side of the curve and a turnbuckle is incorporated into the cast. As the turnbuckle is shortened the curve is further corrected.

casting is a result of the implementation of the Hueter-Volkmann principle. The disadvantages of this form of correction are:

1. Casts must be changed frequently.
2. Since treatment may continue for many years until full bone growth is reached (15+1 years in girls and 17+1 years in boys), casts must be worn for many years.
3. Since most casts cannot be removed at home, they deny the patient personal hygienic and athletic activities.
4. Upon ultimate removal of the cast, the prolonged period of limited activity imposed by casting may lead to loss of muscle and ligamentous tone.
5. Although cast treatment can correct a significant amount of the scoliosis and maintain this correction throughout the use of the cast, a great loss of correction occurs upon removal. (However, progression of scoliosis is at least prevented, which is one of the objectives of treatment.)

Metal and leather molded braces and cast-like molded plastic splints function in the same manner as a plaster cast but permit removal for bathing and exercises. Their disadvantages are the expense for the initial construction and the subsequent modification to accommodate growth and the changes in the scoliosis. Most braces do not correct as well as casts, since they do not have the same contact pressure as the plaster casts. However, they have the advantage of permitting exercise, thus decreasing loss of muscle and ligamentous tone.

Kinetic Correction: Milwaukee Brace

A kinetic form of brace correction is currently exemplified by the Milwaukee brace (Fig. 40). This is a custom-built brace that embodies pelvic support and static correction of the rotatory deformities such as rib angulation and pelvic rotation. Cervical distraction against the occipital pad elongates the

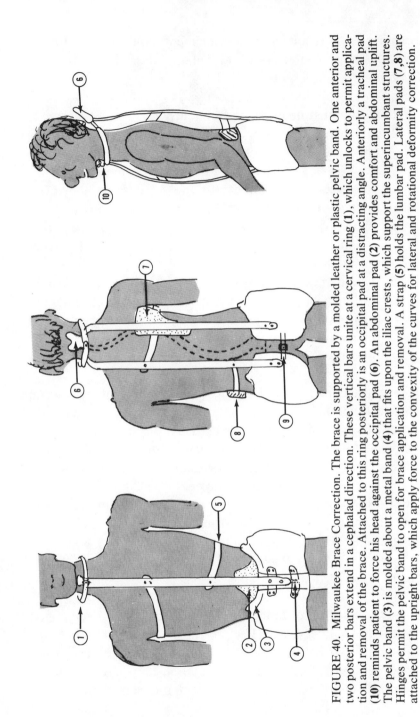

FIGURE 40. Milwaukee Brace Correction. The brace is supported by a molded leather or plastic pelvic band. One anterior and two posterior bars extend in a cephalad direction. These vertical bars unite at a cervical ring (1), which unlocks to permit application and removal of the brace. Attached to this ring posteriorly is an occipital pad at a distracting angle. Anteriorly a tracheal pad (10) reminds patient to force his head against the occipital pad (6). An abdominal pad (2) provides comfort and abdominal uplift. The pelvic band (3) is molded about a metal band (4) that fits upon the iliac crests, which support the superincumbant structures. Hinges permit the pelvic band to open for brace application and removal. A strap (5) holds the lumbar pad. Lateral pads (7,8) are attached to the upright bars, which apply force to the convexity of the curves for lateral and rotational deformity correction.

68

spine and by traction decreases the curves (Fig. 41). The lateral pads tend to prevent further lateral curving and rotation by a restraining pressure (Fig. 42). It is conceivable that these pads also exert corrective passive forces but restraint of progression of curves is their more probable effect (Fig. 43). Thus, all that can be expected of these lateral pads is that they hold curves, not necessarily correct them. In addition to the corrective forces applied by the brace, exercises that increase corrective forces are done actively within the brace. These exercises tend to "pull" the convexity away from one pad and "push" the

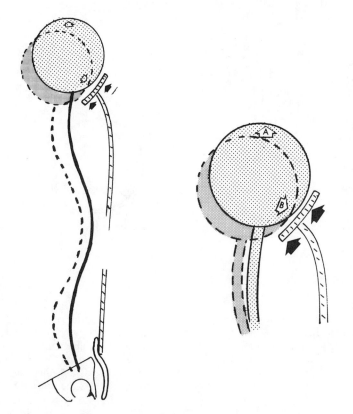

FIGURE 41. Concept of Cervical-Occipital Distraction. On the **right**, the head angles cephalad (**A**) as the patient voluntarily pushes it back against the occipital pad (**B**). This causes the patient to be "taller" and the cervical as well as the lumbar lordosis to decrease (**left**).

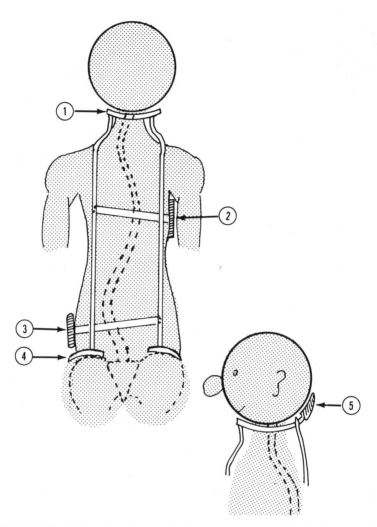

FIGURE 42. Milwaukee Brace Principle. **1** is the occipital ring to which is attached the occipital pad (**5**) and the anterior tracheal pad. **2** is the lateral thoracic pad that presses against the thoracic convexity; patients are taught exercises that tend to pull the convexity away from this pad. **3** is the lumbar correcting pad that presses against the lumbar convexity. **4** illustrates the principle of the "perch" of the pelvic band that supports the upright bars.

concavity toward the opposing pad. Derotation is also attempted in combination with motion toward the midline (Fig. 44). Exercises are also done out of the brace through the range of motion that is otherwise prevented by the brace. The brace is con-

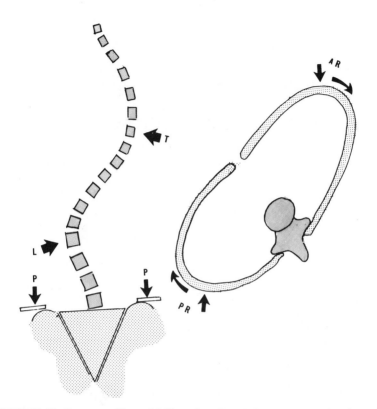

FIGURE 43. Pressure Sites of Milwaukee Brace. **P** represents the sites of perch with downward pressure against the iliac crests. These points are those of the pelvic band. The posterior lateral pads connect to the upright bars that correct or hold the lateral curves and the rotational deformity; they press laterally at the thoracic spine (**T**) and laterally at the lumbar spine (**L**). In the figure on the **right** the anterior rotatory pressure sites (**AR**) and the scapular posterior sites (**PR**) are shown from above. These are the sites away from or toward which the exercises are done.

structed so that it is adjustable to curve changes of the scoliosis and to height growth and change in weight of the child. These braces are made upon a plaster positive mold made from a cast accurately applied to the patient. The positive mold is poured into the cast, which is then bivalved and removed; the brace is then made upon this mold.

The advantages of the Milwaukee brace are:

1. The child is able to remove the brace for toilet and

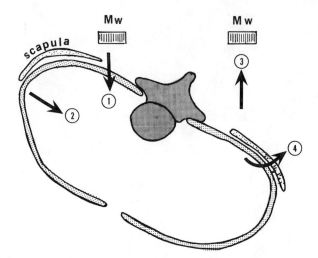

FIGURE 44. Exercises Done in Milwaukee Brace to Decrease Rotation. The posterior upright bars of the brace (**Mw**) are the points against and away from which the child is taught to exercise. The hump of the rib cage (**2**) is "pulled away" from the bar (**1**), and the spine is shifted toward the midline. On the concave side the ribs are pressed toward the bar (**3**) and the entire rib cage is rotated toward that bar (**4**).

shower-bathing activities and for daily one-hour periods to permit exercise activities such as swimming.

2. Lateral and rotatory deformities are actively corrected by performance of specific exercises within the brace that enhance the passive corrective forces of the brace pads.

3. The brace permits almost unlimited activities, excluding only contact sports for the safety of other children and very active sports such as tumbling on a trampoline, horseback riding, and strenuous gymnastics for the safety of the patient.

4. Because of all the physical activities encouraged in and out of the brace, muscle and ligamentous tone is maintained after the brace is ultimately removed.

The disadvantages of the Milwaukee brace are:

1. The brace must be worn day and night (23 out of 24 hours) until full growth, as revealed by x-ray views, is achieved. This usually takes years.

2. The brace, which has some undesirable cosmetic features, must be acceptable to the patient for constant wearing.
3. The patient must agree to daily exercises within the brace.
4. Little correction can be promised or expected. Upon removal of the brace by gradual weaning, much of the correction is frequently lost, but the curve only reverts to its original degree. (If originally the curve was minor and deformity minimal, treatment is obviously "successful.")

The value of the Milwaukee brace, then, lies primarily in maintenance of the current curve status and the prevention of further progression. Various authors have claimed correction of scoliosis of both the lateral curves and rotational deformities, but this correction is minimal and in my personal observation not significant. Prevention of progression, however, of both lateral curving and especially rotational deformity are extremely desirable and justify the use of the Milwaukee brace.

When epiphyseal growth is completed as evidenced by x-ray confirmation and no progression has been noted in recent months, the brace may be gradually withdrawn. The patient is weaned from wearing the brace by removal for varying periods during the day.

The rapidity of the weaning process varies with the doctor, the course of the patient's scoliosis, the severity of the curve, and the dependability of the patient. The brace may be removed for one hour daily with x-rays taken within three months. Progression of the scoliosis may require resumption of wearing the brace full time. Maintenance of the correction may encourage further "weaning."

When stability of the scoliosis has been demonstrated after the patient has been out of the brace eight hours daily, it is usually permissible to continue wearing of the brace at night only for six to twelve months. During the process of weaning frequent x-ray measurement of degree of curve (Cobb method) and degree of rotation (measured by any acceptable method) must be ensured. Whenever loss of correction is noted resumption of brace wearing may be necessary. This is psychologically traumatic and occasionally rejected by the patient who is now a self-conscious adolescent. It is discouraging to the patient and the family that "hard gained" correction from years of wearing a brace has been "lost."

Loss of correction also creates a therapeutic challenge of whether to resume the brace, if so, for how long, or to decide upon operative correction. The latter decision raises the question in the patient's mind of the advisability of wearing a brace in the first place. The use of a Milwaukee brace in early minimal scoliosis ensures that the patient reaches adulthood with minimal cosmetic deformity and a straight, well-balanced spine with good muscle ligamentous tone.

The prescription of the Milwaukee brace can be indicated in any early scoliosis that is progressing and approaching 20° of curvature. In a young child with 10 to 15° curvature and no rotation, the brace can be delayed so long as repeated x-ray examinations are taken every three months. As soon as there is indication of approximately 5° of progression, the brace should be considered.

In a curve of less than 15 to 20° with any noticeable rib angulation or rotation attributable to the thoracic scoliosis, bracing should be considered. Curves of 20°, with or without rotation, are candidates for bracing.

Curves that exceed 50° are poor candidates for the Milwaukee brace unless merely preventing further progression of the curve is the treatment objective and the patient refuses other forms of correction. A curve of that magnitude (50°) is difficult to fit, and since flexibility may be limited, correction is also limited. Pulmonary studies have revealed that the brace apparently results in some respiratory impairment during its wearing by patients with curves that exceed 50°. Curves of that magnitude are best considered for surgical care.

When the major curve is present in the lumbar area, the

Milwaukee brace is markedly limited in its value. Since there are no skeletal points of compression or correction pressures, the brace is effective principally to elongate the spine and correct lumbar lordosis by pelvic tilting from the pelvic band or by distraction from the occipital pad. Exercises away from the posterolateral lumbar pad are of value.

In upper thoracic curves, above T_4 and T_5, brace correction is also difficult since this portion of the spine is removed from direct corrective forces of the brace by the scapular tissues. Traction from the occipital pad has some limited benefit to these curves. Surgery is indicated when the upper thoracic curve progresses and threatens pulmonary or neurological embarrassment.

Where there is rib angulation with potential deformity and curves associated with kyphosis of a significant degree the Milwaukee brace is very effective. Under these conditions, early application is encouraged since rib deformities are better able to be controlled than corrected. Kyphosis responds to the brace in a very short period of time (10 to 14 months) compared with the time it takes for rotatory scoliosis to respond.

Exercises within Brace. Excercises done within the brace are given to the patient as soon as the brace has been fitted and the patient begins wearing it. *Just as exercises alone are of limited value in either correcting or controlling scoliosis, applying a Milwaukee brace without exercises is of limited value.* The effectiveness of a Milwaukee brace depends on its constant wearing (23 out of every 24 hours) and daily exercises performed in and out of the brace.

When the decision is made to prescribe a Milwaukee brace, it must be with full acceptance by the patient—not merely upon the insistence of the parents and/or the physician. The child must also be informed of the necessity of continuous wearing and simultaneous exercises and must accept and cooperate. To insist on a brace for a reluctant or resistant child who also will fail to exercise or wear the brace, is an exercise in futility.

It is desirable for the patient for whom a brace is prescribed to be under periodic care of a specially trained physical therapist. The therapist instructs in the exercises, supervises them so that they will be done properly and for the duration of the brace wearing, and modifies them as the curvature dictates. By becoming a friend to the child, as well as a member of the therapeutic team, the therapist is in an excellent position to evaluate the emotional reaction of the child and the parents to the entire program. Problems of clothing, sitting comfort, school and physical-education activities, social activities, etc., raise questions that can be answered by a trained and interested therapist.

Not only must the patient be seen at periodic intervals, but the brace must also be checked for possible adjustments. This is done at meetings of the "team," (approximately every three to four months), which consists of the patient and her brace, the parents, the supervising physician, the therapist, and the orthotist. Special clinics for scoliosis patients are desirable, since they allow to be present at a single session members who can share similar experiences and solutions to minor problems.

The exercises should preferably be taught to the patient before the brace is procured and must be initiated as a daily practice immediately upon the acquisition and wearing of the brace.

Scoliosis exercises are of two types. The standard conditioning type is done in and out of the brace and is intended to maintain the strength of the trunk muscles, which may be restricted by the use of the brace (Fig. 45). These exercises are aimed at strengthening the abdominal muscles and stressing proper posture. Within the brace, all athletic activities other than violent gymnastics and contact sports are encouraged.

The other specific type of exercise includes those meant to decrease the major curves (Fig. 45). These exercises are aimed at (1) Decreasing lumbar lordosis, (2) reducing the thoracic (rib) hump, and (3) forcing out the thoracic depression on the contralateral aspect of the hump. To do these, the patient

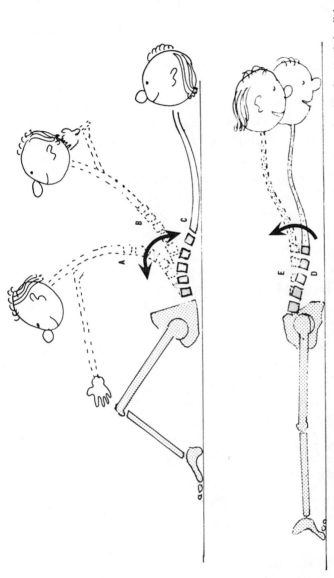

FIGURE 45. Exercises: Abdominal and Extension. The **top** figure depicts abdominal exercises of value for "pelvic tilting" to flatten the lumbar lordosis. For patients with weak abdominal muscles, starting position **A** is preferable. The lumbar spine is flexed and the arms extended to place the hands near the knees should the trunk lean back too far. The exercise is to gradually and rhythmically go from position **A** to **B** and ultimately to **C**. These reversed *sitting up* exercises strengthen the abdominal flexors. The **bottom** figure shows the extension exercises to decrease the thoracic kyphosis. They should not simultaneously hyperextend the lumbar lordosis (**D** to **E**). Simultaneously the scapula should be adducted to extend the upper spine.

"pulls away" from the pad over the hump and presses forward toward the brace-bar side. A pelvic tilting exercise is practiced to decrease the lordosis (Fig. 46).

Traction within the brace is attempted by what can be termed *distraction*. The patient forces the head back against the occipital pad and attempts to get "taller." Distraction exercises can be taught with the therapist or the parents pushing down on the vertex of the patient's head while he "pushes up" to "get taller." This exercise aligns the head over the pelvis, decreases the cervical lordosis and the dorsal kyphosis, and also "tilts" the pelvis, thus decreasing the lumbar lordosis. This is an excellent postural exercise done in and out of the brace. It can be done by the patient alone if he places a 2- to 10-pound sandbag on top of his head for frequent 10- to 30-minute periods during the day (Fig. 47).

"Round-Back" Bracing. In children with "round back" deformity that is considered to be of pathological significance, treatment with the Milwaukee brace is of great value. The same scoliosis Milwaukee brace is constructed for the patient, but the pad is placed posteriorly and horizontally between the two

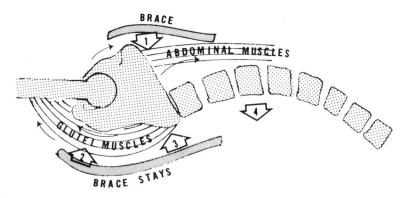

FIGURE 46. "Pelvic Tilting": Brace and Exercise. To decrease the lumbar lordosis, the lumbosacral angle (**L-S**) must be decreased. This is accomplished by the upward pull of the abdominal muscles upon the anterior pelvis and the downward pull of the gluteal muscles on the posterior pelvis. The brace assists the muscles and maintains the tilted pelvis. **1**, **2**, and **3** are points of contact of the brace that serve to decrease lordosis (**4**).

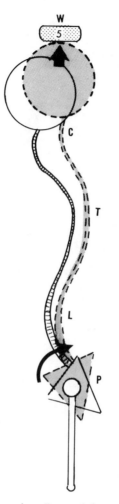

FIGURE 47. Distraction Exercise. By applying a weight (**W**) of 2 to 10 pounds (sandbag) on the head for varying periods during the day (10 to 30 minutes), the cervical lordosis (**C**) is decreased and ultimately the lumbar lordosis (**L**) also decreases. This *distraction* principle is employed in the Milwaukee brace. This exercise is also valuable to teach proper erect posture.

posterior bars at the level just slightly below the apical vertebra of the kyphosis (Fig. 48).

Exercises perscribed for Milwaukee brace treatment of kyphosis "round back" or the kyphosis associated with

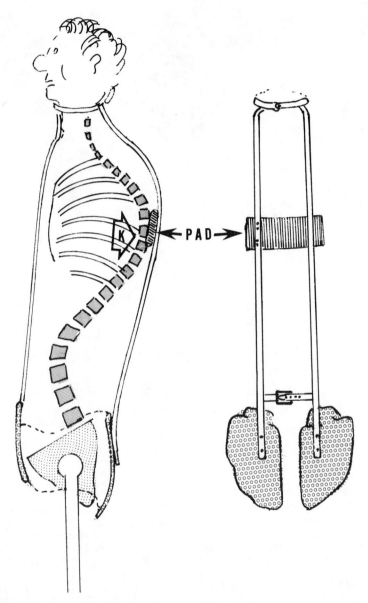

FIGURE 48. Modified Milwaukee Brace for "Round Back." The Milwaukee brace for excessive dorsal kyphosis (**K**) has the same pelvis portion as the scoliosis apparatus; but in addition it has a horizontal pad placed posteriorly that presses against the apical vertebra. The occipital ring is identical to that of the scoliosis brace. Exercises done in this brace differ slightly from those done in the scoliosis brace.

scoliosis are identical to those for scoliosis with the addition of extension and hyperextension exercises of the thoracic spine. Pectoral muscle stretching exercises, "flat" neck exercises to decrease cervical lordosis and scapular adduction exercises can be added with benefit.

In the round back posture where scapular forward rotation, not the thoracic vertebral kyphosis, is not the major deforming condition, exercise can be beneficial. When there is structural vertebral kyphosis, exercises alone are of no significant value and kyphosis or round back will persist and probably progress. There is no medical harm that results from excessive round back that makes treatment mandatory. However, concern on the part of the patient and/or her parents about uncosmetic appearance may initiate the use of a brace.

As the years progress marked dorsal kyphosis causes gradual impairment of shoulder range of motion and because of resulting compensatory cervical lordosis may precipitate symptomatic cervical diskogenic disease. In adult kyphosis when epiphyseal closure has occurred, neither brace nor exercise will improve the dorsal curve.

There are many early minor curves that could well be benefitted by wearing a Milwaukee brace, but parents delay in acquiring the brace because of cost only to realize upon subsequent examination that progression has occurred. There also are curves (scoliosis) in young age groups that might require bracing during sleeping hours only, but which may ultimately require daytime use also as well. In these patients when the future is not predictable, the decision is frequently made not to recommend a brace, only to be regretted later when there has been progression.

To obviate delay in procuring the current expensive appliance, a brace of different construction and material, of much lower cost, and less difficult to construct would be desirable. Such a brace would ensure early application that, if later found unnecessary, would not have caused a financial hardship to the family. Recently a premolded plastic pelvic shell resembling the Milwaukee pelvis portion of the brace has been made which can be quickly modified (in 2 hours) to contour the patient and have the other brace elements added. Besides the minimal cost, the rapidity of construction and its easy alterations for growth make this brace a possible replacement for the current Milwaukee brace.

In early curves of less than 20° wearing a Milwaukee brace only during hours of sleep and daily exercises is being advocated. This approach is intended to supercede that of "waiting out" and observing the scoliosis until there is evidence of progression, the earliest manifestation of which is a beginning of a tendency of the scoliosis toward rib rotation deformity. In many cases the presence of mild rib protrusion and a curve of 20° is not correctable, but early bracing would have prevented progression and resulted in an acceptable scoliosis.

Traction

Traction has been used for centuries in treatment of scoliosis. Methods have included hanging, bed rest with horizontal traction, and preoperative traction before cast application. This latter method of traction is applied on a Risser type frame. Elongation is admittedly of temporary value.

Cotrel's Method. Recently Cotrel has devised a method that utilizes traction applied by weights and force exerted by the patient's leg to the degree that it can be tolerated by the patient (Fig. 49). Cotrel advocates exercises to be done in conjunction with traction. These exercises are similar to those given to patients wearing the Milwaukee brace. Cotrel's traction has been advocated for continuous night use and varying periods during the daytime. There is no concomitant wearing of a brace. This form of treatment has not been used long, and its value is not yet established. However, it is known to have value when used preoperatively and followed by use of a specially designed table upon which patient undergoes surgery while in traction (Fig. 50).

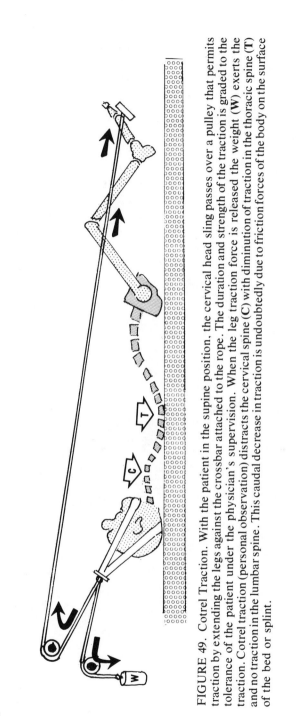

FIGURE 49. Cotrel Traction. With the patient in the supine position, the cervical head sling passes over a pulley that permits traction by extending the legs against the crossbar attached to the rope. The duration and strength of the traction is graded to the tolerance of the patient under the physician's supervision. When the leg traction force is released the weight (W) exerts the traction. Cotrel traction (personal observation) distracts the cervical spine (C) with diminution of traction in the thoracic spine (T) and no traction in the lumbar spine. This caudal decrease in traction is undoubtedly due to friction forces of the body on the surface of the bed or splint.

83

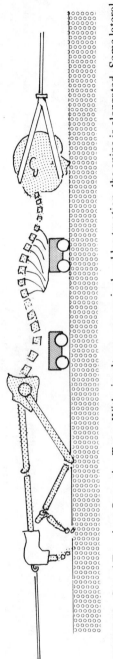

FIGURE 50. Cotrel Traction: Operative Type. With simultaneous cervical and leg traction, the spine is elongated. Some lateral curve correction also results. The wheeled supports allow traction while decreasing body friction against the table. Surgery can be performed in this apparatus.

Cephalopelvic. This type of traction plus localized lateral pads in a traction frame facilitate correction of scoliosis for ultimate casting or surgery. Cotrel slings suspended from the frame bars also are efficient to partially derotate the deformity prior to casting or surgery (see Figure 51).

Halo-Pelvic. In severe scoliosis, of various causes, halo-

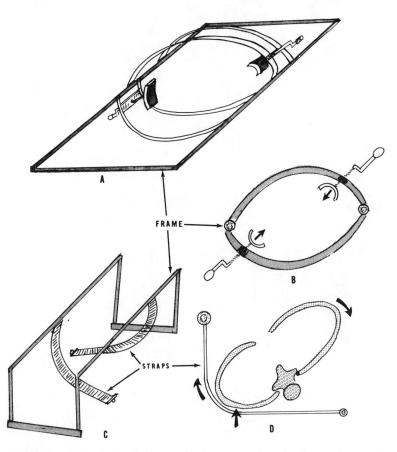

FIGURE 51. Frame Scoliosis Correction. **A** depicts the frame commonly called a *Risser frame*. The rounded pads on a crank swivel are placed against the convexity of the curve and pressure is applied to rerotate the curve. **B** is a side view of the Risser-type frame. The arrows depict the corrective forces. **C** is a Cotrel-type frame with lateral rotatory corrective forces applied by straps. **D** depicts the forces acting upon the rib deformity. The straight arrow is the pressure against the "rib hump." The curved arrow is the corrective rotatory force direction.

femoral or halo-pelvic traction has been employed. The halo is applied directly to the head with pin fixation to the skull. The femoral counter traction is applied through pins inserted through the distal femurs. Weights are applied in small increments approaching 30 pounds on the head and 15 pounds on

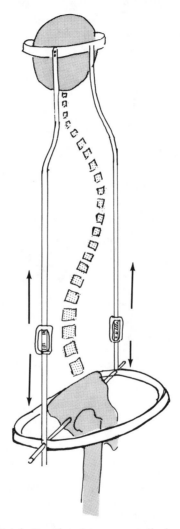

FIGURE 52. Halo-Pelvic Traction. In severe scoliosis a halo is pinned to the skull and a pelvic band to ilia of the pelvis. Upright bars connect the two bands, and as they are elongated the spine is also elongated and scoliosis corrected. Traction is continuous and permits ambulation of the patient.

each leg. Maximum correction is considered to have occurred in three weeks, although currently Japanese orthopaedists advocate this traction for several months. Obviously bed confinement must be used for this type of traction.

Surgery is performed after two to three weeks of halo-femoral traction. After surgical connection with or without internal instrumentation, a cast incorporating the halo apparatus is applied for nine months or more.

A halo-pelvic hoop apparatus has more recently been devised that permits traction and also allows ambulation (Fig. 52). By its pelvic fixation the stress and possible injury to the hip joints that occasionally results from halo-femoral traction is minimized (Fig. 53).

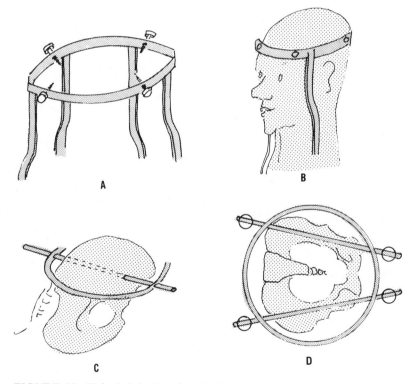

FIGURE 53. Halo-Pelvic Traction Devices. A depicts the halo with skull screws that fits about the skull (B). C shows the pin inserted through the ilium of the pelvis that is then fitted to the pelvic band (D).

The pelvic hoop portion of the apparatus is held by rods that penetrate the iliac crests. Upright bars to these rods ascend and are connected to the halo to cause distraction forces upon the scoliosis. This traction is maintained longer than the halo-femoral traction once it is seen that surgery is also possible within the apparatus.

SURGICAL TREATMENT OF SCOLIOSIS

Although surgical correction techniques are beyond the scope of this monograph, it behooves the interested physician or therapist to have a basic understanding of the indication for surgery, some of the current techniques, their indications, contraindications, and possible complications. To better discuss surgical intervention with the patient and his family, knowledge of surgical procedures is very desirable.

Indications

Indications for recommending surgical treatment rather than nonsurgical conservative treatment may be enumerated as follows:

1. The patient has been under brace treatment and, in spite of good brace care has progressed in his scoliosis.
2. The patient is seen too late in the course of his illness for brace treatment. "Too late" implies that he has a thoracic curve of over 50°, an unacceptably deforming curve that can only be "held" by bracing without hope of correction, or that he is a child with completed or nearly completed vertebral growth (girls with bone age 15 or boys with bone age 17).
3. Surgery is indicated for a patient with a thoracic curve over 50° even though they may be cosmetically acceptable to him. Curves over 50° have increased morbidity and mortality, and even after completion of vertebral growth

can and usually do increase in their curvature. Vital capacity tends to diminish in curves over 60°.

4. The patient has intractable pain that can be attributed to or is related to scoliosis.
5. Surgery is recommended for the patient who is laterally "decompensated" with the occiput not over the sacrum by a significant degree and whose scoliosis is not being "held." A decompensated scoliosis (unbalanced) has a propensity for progression even with adequate bracing.
6. The patient experiences psychological decompensation to the scoliosis deformity.

Procedures

When surgery has been decided upon by the physician and recommended to the patient, the choice of surgical procedure must be decided. What criteria decide the type of preoperative treatment necessary and the method of surgery depends upon the experience of the surgeon. Some generalities can be made from the literature and from the experience of the author.

Harrington Rods. In curves of less than 60°, instrumentation using Harrington rods may be employed without preoperative correction by casting or by recumbent traction. Curves that exceed 60° with or without flexibility may be benefitted by preoperative traction. The type of traction and duration depends again on the experience of the surgeon. In curves exceeding 90° many surgeons advocate preoperative halo-femoral traction. The type of scoliosis also dictates the method of surgery and the preoperative treatment. Procedures vary among geographical areas as well as from clinic to clinic so that no "standard" procedure can be advocated. Hopefully some day, as is anticipated by the Scoliosis Research Society, standards will evolve as guidelines, and a register of competent surgeons with expertise in scoliosis will be available in generalized regions of the world for consultation and care.

Currently the extent of surgical intervention is postulated to include in the length of the fusion "all vertebrae rotated into the convexity of the major curve and one vertebra above and one vertebra below."[1] Preoperative traction may derotate one or more vertebrae, thus shortening the extent of fusion. In a single major curve all the vertebrae in the curve plus one proximal and one distal are usually fused. If there is a compensatory lumbar curve to balance the thoracic, only the thoracic curve is fused (Fig. 54). The lumbar curve may need treatment, either surgical or nonsurgical if much growth remains.

In a lumbosacral curve that is decompensated with a nonstructural compensatory thoracic curve, correction may be achieved by centering L_4 over the pelvis and fusing. Double major curves that require surgery require that both curves be fused.

Surgical fusion may be performed through a window cut out of the plaster body cast. Internal fixation correction by a rod is considered more effective in that more correction can be gained and maintained than by external correction (Fig. 55).

Other surgical procedures may be employed to increase the surgical benefits. Among these procedures are the surgical "release" of the costotransverse ligaments of the concave side of the curve. Osteotomy of the transverse processor on the convex side also decreases the rib "hump" deformity; merely lateral correction does not. Some rotatory correction is achieved by merely correcting the convexity, but this correction is more evident in the lumbar region and decreases as the curve goes more cephalad in the thoracic region. High thoracic vertebrae derotate little, if any, with Harrington instrumentation.

Opinions vary regarding the advisability of using compression rods on the convex side in conjunction with distraction rods on the concave side. Many authorities do not feel that compression rods increase the correction and may even make fusion on the convex side more different.

In most surgical procedures, casting is used postoperatively. When precasting has been utilized, the same cast that has been

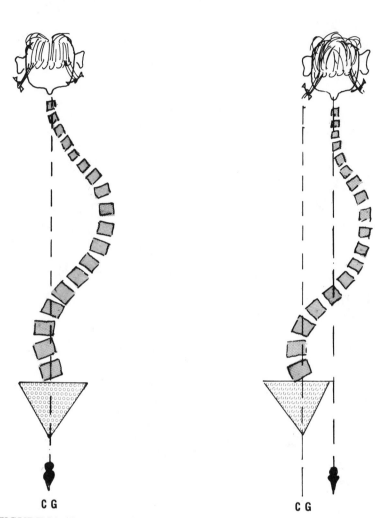

C G   C G

FIGURE 54. Compensated Scoliosis. The scoliosis in the figure on the left is well balanced with the occipital vertex directly above the sacrum. All superincumbent curves return the head to balance above the center of gravity (CG). When the scoliosis is decompensated the spine is unbalanced with the head lateral to the center of gravity as shown in the right figure. A deviation of 2 to 3 centimeters places abnormal stress against the spine and aggravates the scoliosis.

either "windowed" over the incision or has been bivalved can be applied postoperatively and a new cast applied two weeks postoperatively.

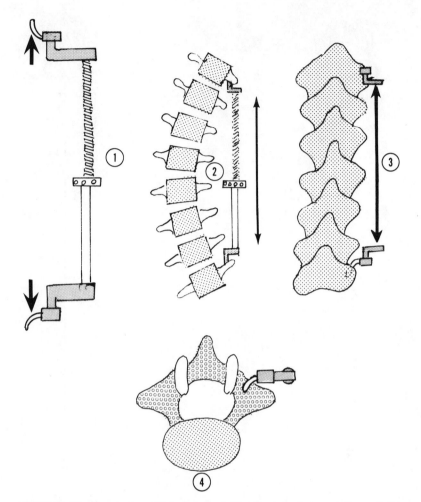

FIGURE 55. Harrington Rod: Internal Fixation. Instrumentation of the Harrington variety (1) elongates the concave side of the curve (2). It veritably "jacks up" the spine (3). 4 depicts the site of rod insertion into the lamina. As the rod elongates, the curves decrease. This instrumentation is followed by operative fusion of the curve.

Postoperative ambulation depends upon the surgeon's experience and decision. It varies from ambulation in two weeks to complete bed rest for one month followed by semi-ambulatory privileges for an additional two months. Casting is usually maintained for 9 to 13 months. Six months after surgery the cast is removed, and x-rays are taken to assess the degree of

92

correction and the status of the fusion. A cast is reapplied for the remainder of time.

After surgical fusion there is an expected loss of correction of 5 to 10°. Some of this loss of correction following successful surgery utilizing instrumentation is attributed to the erosion of bone at the hook sites. A postoperative Milwaukee brace is claimed to release the load upon the rod hooks.

Dwyer Procedure. A surgical anterior approach with cable traction reduction has been advocated by Dwyer[2] (Fig. 56).

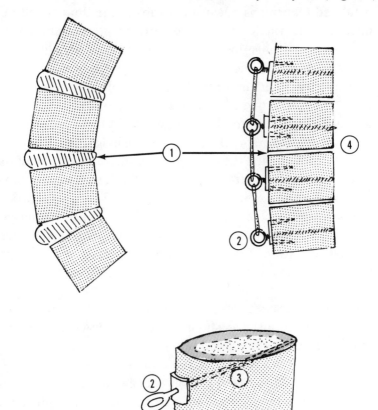

FIGURE 56. Dwyer Procedure. The intervertebral disks (1) are removed between all the vertebrae included in the major scoliosis curves. Dwyer staples (2) are inserted into the vertebrae. Screws transverse the entire body (3) of the vertebrae, then cables connect to each staple. Shortening the cable on the convex side of the curve straightens the spine (4).

Correction is dramatic and has increasingly more advocates; but it is technically more difficult, and long-term results are not yet available. The intervertebral disks included in the curve are removed as are the cartilage end-plates allowing more curve correction and fusion of the decorticated vertebrae. The major benefit of this procedure is gained in thoracolumbar and lumbar curves. This procedure is *not* recommended for high thoracic curves because of the surgical technical difficulty. Mid or lower thoracic curves do not correct as well as lumbar curves. It is postulated that this is because the ribs in the thoracic curves impeded vertebral derotation and thoracic intervertebral disks are smaller and thus do not permit much later mobility.

Complications of the Dwyer Procedure are those of major chest surgery. Interruption of the intercostal blood vessels may impair the cord blood supply. Improperly placed screws into the bodies have reportedly damaged the spinal cord. Screws incompletely traversing the body may dislodge, thus eliminating their traction pinch. Because of the anterior position of the cable, many patients treated with the Dwyer procedure have developed a marked increase in kyphosis. The Dwyer procedure is not advocated in severe osteoporosis since the screws and plate will not remain imbedded in the vertebral bodies. Because of these numerous complications and technical difficulties, many surgeons are not yet advocating this procedure.

All surgical procedures and major nonoperative procedures have complications that should be made known to potential patients. These complications must also be known by the treating physician who must anticipate them to prevent them. In addition to possible complications specific to scoliosis, all general surgical complications such as anesthetic complication, blood type incompatibilities, blood transfusion, and transfer of hepatitis are also possible in operative treatment of scoliosis. Complications specific to scoliosis have been discussed and include neurological complications and failure of fusion (pseudoarthrosis); pseudoarthrosis may require reoperating.

Postoperative care of the scoliosis patient requires excessive care in returning the patient from the operating table to the bed. Staff, team-coordinated effort is required. Smooth anesthetic recovery must be ensured to avoid jerky movements and uncontrolled coughing. Before moving the patient, it is desirable that the patient be aware so that the neurological status of her lower extremities can be determined. Coughing exercises are preferably *not* started during the first 24 hours, but breathing exercises should be started within the first few days. Surgeons vary in their opinions regarding "rolling over" by the patient, whether unassisted or aided by attendants, but it appears to be universally accepted that patient should *not* sit up until the cast has been applied. Ambulation with the cast is started in the first week of wearing in some clinics and only after many weeks of wearing elsewhere. No standard procedure has been established. A brace or cast may be worn from six months to one year.

Admittedly, postoperative complications are rare, but they are possible and should be weighted carefully by the patient, the family, and the physician. Since treatment (operative or nonoperative) in many cases of scoliosis is undertaken because of cosmetic rather than life-saving concerns, it is all the more necessary that possible complications be discussed with the patient. Not only has the need for transfusions increased the possibility of effects of blood incompatibilities and hepatitis transfer, but the duration of the surgery, often accompanied by a moderate loss of blood, may cause shock. Pressure sores can occur due to the external pressure of the corrective casts. Excessive cervical traction may cause brachial plexus damage or cranial VI nerve palsy. Rapid elongation of the vertebral column by instrumentation can cause cord damage with resultant paresis or paralysis. Cord trauma is always a possible surgical complication in any vertebral column surgery. Gluteal artery injury has been reported at the bone donor site in the iliac crest.

The "cast syndrome" (Fig. 57) is a rare but serious

95

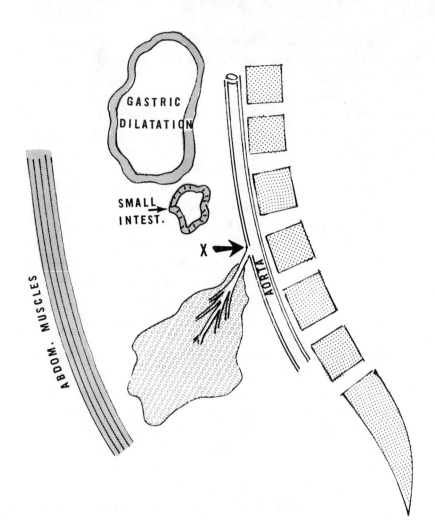

FIGURE 57. Cast Syndrome. Servere ileus occurs as a result of distension of the stomach and abdominal contents. The duodenum is compressed between the superior mesenteric artery anteriorly and the aorta and vertebral column posteriorly. The lumbar lordosis is supposedly increased, which increases traction upon major blood vessels and increases the arterial angle (**X**), obstructing both the mesenteric vein and mesenteric artery. The abdominal muscles become totally ineffective in decreasing the lordosis or the distention.

complication. The syndrome is also medically termed the *superior mesentery artery syndrome* and may result from application of a body plaster jacket. This is a syndrome consisting of severe ileus with metabolic imbalance and severe alkalosis. The cause is considered to be distention and compression of the duodenum between the superior mesenteric artery anteriorly and the aorta and vertebral column posteriorly. The ligament of Treitz immobilizes the fourth portion of the duodenum. Treatment is to correct medically the alkalosis and to release the ileus by nasogastric suction with or without removal of the cast. When ileus is very severe, duodenojejunostomy or gastrojejunostomy may be necessary.

When one considers the many surgical difficulties and complications of operative treatment of scoliosis, the need for early recognition and early nonoperative treatment becomes more evident.

Since scoliosis is more frequent in children and treatment is psychologically traumatic to both the child and the parents, sympathetic understanding and care are important. The many years involved in brace treatment, cast treatment, and preoperative and postoperative care require careful judgment in diagnosis and treatment, as well as thorough, patient discussions with everyone concerned.

The probability of unacceptable cosmetic appearance resulting from scoliosis may be the only indication for further diagnostic procedures or treatment. This may not be apparent to the patient or may be frightening to the parents. This is understandable, and the feelings of the patient and her family toward diagnosis and treatment must be fully discussed with them in understandable terms. The financial cost of scoliosis treatment, whether bracing or surgical, is also significant and must be given consideration in such discussions. Ultimately, the psychological effect on an adolescent girl that results from the wearing of a bulky brace that cannot fully be concealed presents social adjustment problems. Occasionally a clinical psychologist may be needed, but usually an attentive, interested physician, a therapist, and an orthotist can manage scoliosis patients well.

References

1. L. A. Goldstein: The surgical treatment of idiopathic scoliosis. *In* Scoliosis, G. C. Robin (Ed.), Academic Press, Inc., New York, 1973, pp. 95–102.
2. A. F. Dwyer, N. C. Newton, and A. A. Sherwood: An anterior approach to scoliosis. A preliminary report. Clin. Orthop. 62:192, 1969.

CHAPTER 7

Adult Scoliosis

After completion of vertebral growth at approximately fifteen years in girls and seventeen in boys any existing scoliosis persists into adult life. The major impairment from this adult scoliosis, as in children, is a cosmetic deformity. In more severe scoliosis exceeding 50° in the thoracic region, cardiopulmonary complications are possible. Large lumbar curves may also become painful.

Confirmation of adult scoliosis is the same as in childhood where clinical examination reveals the site and extent of lateral and rotatory curving and x-ray confirms the degree, site, and cause of the scoliosis. The vertebral body deformation can now be compared to the intervertebral disk space symmetry.

Treatment of adult scoliosis is different from that of the childhood curves. The adult spine is less flexible and thus less reversible (correctable) by elimination of gravity, flexibility exercises, bracing or casting, and is less amenable to operative correction. Progression of adult scoliosis is not a result of vertebral epiphyseal deformation, but of asymmetrical intervertebral disk compression and degeneration on the concave side of the curves. Increase in adult scoliosis due to the disk deterioration has been said to equal 1° per year. A scoliosis of 45° upon completion of vertebral growth could be considered acceptable, but within 20 years, curves of patients then in their mid thirties could theoretically approach 65°. This extent of progression is not usual.

Treatment has usually been that of weight reduction, active and passive exercises, or bracing or corsetting to support the spine if pain occurs. The benefit of nonoperative methods has not been documented, and thus the value of this kind of treatment has not been established. Improvement of pulmonary function by nonoperative treatment has been studied, and it has been found that it does *not* occur.

More recently there has been an international trend to consider operative intervention of adult scoliosis. The standard methods of preoperative care, such as bracing, casting, traction, and halo-pelvic traction, have all been used. Operative procedures of internal fixation and correction and the Dwyer procedure also have their advocates.

Results of surgery for adult scoliosis are not yet documented. Improvement of 50% in a 65° curve has questionable cosmetic value even with rib osteotomy. When surgical treatment of adult scoliosis is seen in the light of its morbidity, its possible complications, and the increase in mortality resulting from its use, its value remains equivocal. No signficant pulmonary function improvement results, so that impairment of pulmonary function as an indication for surgical intervention remains vague. Further improvement in surgical techniques, better criteria for recognizing indications, and controlled studies may change the current surgical concept and experience.

Scoliosis alone is not the cause of a higher incidence of low back pain in patients under the age of sixty. With further aging, however, and concomitant degenerative changes in the spine, symptoms attributable to foraminal closure and neural compression can occur. The foraminal closure is caused by degenerative arthropathy of the facets and marginal osteophytes (Fig. 58).Thickening of the lamina and the ligamentous flavum also contribute to the foraminal closure.

Neural compression causes radicular pain, weakness and

100

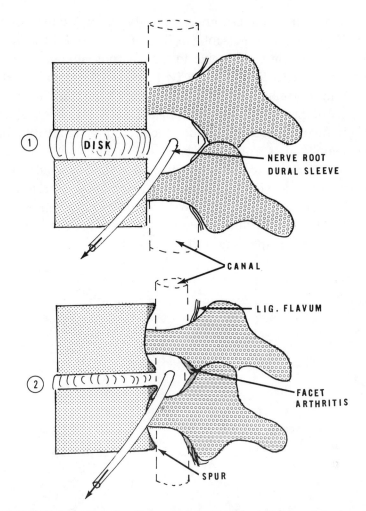

FIGURE 58. Degenerative Changes of the Vertebral Column. 1 depicts the normal functional units of the vertebral column. 2 shows that with disk degeneration the vertebral bodies approximate as do the pedicles and the posterior facets. Osteoarthritic spurs develop, facets undergo osteoarthrosis, and the ligamentum flavum thickens. These changes narrow the intervertebral foramina and the spinal canal.

atrophy of the involved myotomes, and sensory changes in the lower extremities. Radicular pain from this foraminal closure is usually unilaterial pain, noted upon standing and walking and relieved by sitting and lying down. When pain becomes intractable and neural changes progress, only surgical intervention can afford relief. In the scoliosis literature, there is little or no reference to pain attributable to lumbar root compression directly related to the scoliosis (Fig. 59). Collis and Ponseti[1] could not correlate severity of low back symptoms with the severity of the spinal curvature. All neurological deficits, either peripheral or central, reported in the literature are attributable to spinal stenosis from other causes (Fig. 60).

When the spinal canal is narrowed and the enclosed neural tissues compromised, symptoms resembling intermittent claudication can result (Fig. 61). Neurological changes can vary from relatively minor ones to those such as root changes, intractable pain, sphincter difficulty, and sexual dysfunction.

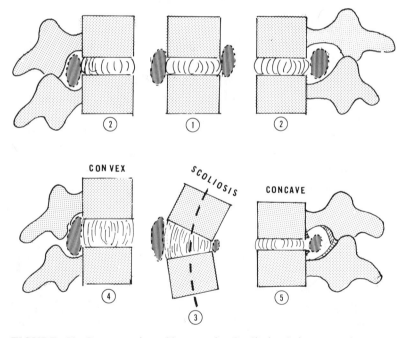

FIGURE 59. Degenerative Changes in Scoliotic Spines. 1 shows an anterior-posterior view of the spine, revealing equal intervertebral foraminal openings (2). In scoliosis (3) on the convex side the foramina open wider (4), and on the concave side (5) the foramina narrow. Degenerative changes such as osteophytes of the vertebral bodies, thickening of the lamina, and posterior facet arthrosis further decrease the foraminal openings.

102

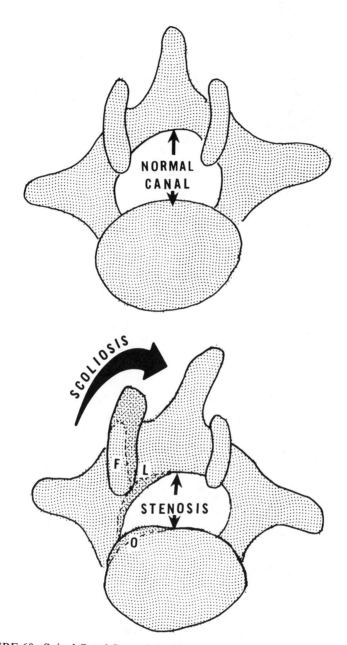

FIGURE 60. Spinal Canal Stenosis in Scoliosis. The deformity that occurs from lateral and rotational forces causes spinal canal stenosis as a result of thickening of the lamina (**L**), osteophytosis of the vertebral bodies (**0**), and thickening of the facets (**F**).

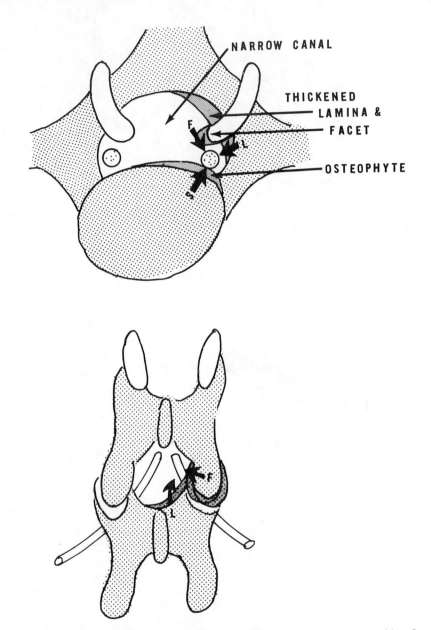

FIGURE 61. Degenerative Changes in Scoliosis. On the concave side of scoliosis curve the lamina thickens (**L**), the facets undergo degenerative changes (**F**), and spurs (**S**) form on the vertebral bodies. These changes decrease the spinal canal width and encroach upon the nerve root and its dural sleeve. Neurological symptoms can result.

104

Conservative treatment is rarely effective. Ultimately treatment requires complete deroofing of the involved area, which may include multiple levels. Surgical treatment may require total laminectomy, foraminotomy, section of the ligamentous flavum and resection of osteoarthritic spurs. Surgery, and therefore accurate diagnosis, may require careful myelography, but when the indications for surgery are clear, decompression is usually beneficial.

Reference

1. D. K. Collis and I. V. Ponseti: Long-term followup of patients with idiopathic scoliosis not treated surgically. J. Bone Joint Surg. 51:425, 1969.

CHAPTER 8

Cardiopulmonary Function

Patients who develop moderate to severe scoliosis with major thoracic deformity have the possibility of cardiac pulmonary complication. Pulmonary complication with secondary cardiac impairment is one of the three reasons given for treating scoliosis. The others are cosmesis and pain.

There is a relationship between the degree and the region of the scoliosis and the impaired pulmonary function. Curves in the thoracic area, both upper and lower or thoracolumbar curves that approach and exceed 50°, are considered candidates for pulmonary embarrassment. In curves in these regions and of this magnitude there is a reduction in vital capacity, total lung capacity, and expiratory peak flow rate. Vital capacity is related inversely to the degree of increasing curvature, but is even more closely correlated to the rotational deformity of the vertebrae involved in the curve. Patients who have paralytic scoliosis such as that seen in post poliomyelitis are impaired further from the associated abdominal and intercostal muscle paresis. In paralytic scoliosis the effort required in increasing the depth of aspiration may be three times that of normal.

Certain concepts of normal cardiopulmonary physiology warrant discussion so that abnormal deviations become meaningful. Vital capacity (VC) is the amount of air the person can

107

expire after maximal inspiration. Inspiratory capacity (IC) is the maximum volume inspired from resting respiratory level, and the expiratory reserve volume (ERV) is the maximum volume expired from resting expiratory level. Residual volume (RV) is the volume of gas in the lungs after maximal expiration as measured at the resting respiratory level. Total lung capacity is the lung volume after maximum inspiration (VC + RV). (See Fig. 62.)

These capacities clinically can be measured by use of a simple bellows-type spirometer. The values reflect the elasticity of the lungs and the efficiency of the respiratory muscles. Chest deformity with rib cage contracture and distortion cause respiratory impairment.

Normal standards are used for comparision and observed

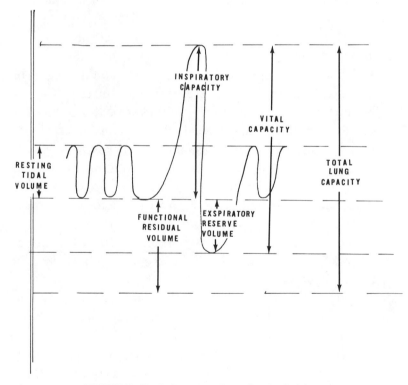

FIGURE 62. Pulmonary Function Definitions.

values and data should be stated in *liters and percentages*. Forced tests are used as standard tests.

Forced vital capacity is vital capacity with expiration as forceful and rapid as possible (FVC). Forced expiratory volume ($FEV_{1.0}$) is the volume of gas expired over a given time interval during FVC. Discrepancy occurs when the standards have been computed with the height of non-scoliotic patients. Stature is decreased in severe scoliosis and thus values are distorted. Lung volumes predicted according to the patient's arm span and height are not accurate in severe scoliosis.

FEV 1.0% normal

Age	♂	♀
20–29	80.1 ± 6.6	80.5 ± 5.3
30–39	75.8 ± 7.4	76.8 ± 5.6
40–49	74.8 ± 6.5	75.7 ± 4.6

Blood-gas level and acid-base balance can also be determined to evaluate pulmonary function, but this is rarely needed in screening early mild scoliosis deformities. Disturbances in blood gases are usually found only in adults with moderately severe scoliosis. Rarely, if ever, are pulmonary problems in children of such severity that they result in alteration of the blood gases. These tests essentially are of value in severely impaired patients and are used preoperatively to prevent anesthetic complications.

Patients with advanced scoliosis may develop a dyspnea with a breathing pattern of frequent, rapid breaths with a small volume of air being moved during a specific period of time. In kyphoscoliosis, the total lung capacity is not uncommonly half of what it should be. It may be below 3.0 L. with normal being 4.0 L. The volume may be as low as 1 L. with simultaneous abnormal arterial gas tensions attributable to alveolar hypoventilation and a disturbed ventilation-perfusion ratio (V/Q).

Breathing may become "strenuous" to the patient because the rib cage, besides being deformed, may be relatively immobile. Patients with kyphoscoliosis have considerable dyspnea on exertion and limited activities for many years before blood gas abnormalities are noted.

Pulmonary hypertension can result from the arterial bed being mechanically restricted leading to cor pulmonale. Cor pulmonale is essentially right ventricular hypertrophy that may progress to cardiac decompensation.

Diagnosis of pulmonary cardiac pathology creating cor pulmonale is made by clinical cardiac auscultation. X-rays may be difficult to interpret because of the deformed rib cage, but the cardiac silhouette and electrocardiogram are helpful diagnostic tools.

All pathological studies have as yet failed to differentiate the pathology or to clarify the pathomechanics of cor pulmonale. Even Xenon studies for determining lung function have failed to reveal abnormalities in ventilation or blood flow in scoliotic children, but have demonstrated some slight impairment in the lower lung fields of adults with scoliosis. Treatment of cor pulmonale with failure is essentially that of treating the cardiac failure.

Routine pulmonary function studies seem to indicate that significant pulmonary impairment occurs in curvatures of 60° or more. After treatment, either operative or nonoperative, no significant change in total lung capacity or vital capacity is noted as a result of treatment. Mean minute ventilation actually has been shown to decrease, but oxygen consumption remains unchanged. Physiologic dead space decreased, but this made *no* change in respiration. Gucker[1] showed that correcting scoliosis by wedging a localized cast produced 21% loss of vital capacity in paralytic scoliosis and 29% in idiopathic scoliosis.

Failure to improve respiration in curves of 50° or more by either operative or nonoperative intervention adds further incentive for early diagnosis and treatment of minimal curves before structural changes cause irreversible respiratory embarrassment. Rotational deformity causes greater respiratory difficulty than lateral curving, and its presence requires even earlier recognition and treatment, bracing, and frequent followup so that surgical intervention may be considered when there is progression of scoliosis in spite of adequate treatment.

Reference

1. T. Gucker, III: Changes in vital capacity in scoliosis: Preliminary reports on effects of treatment. J. Bone Joint Surg. [Am.] 44:469, 1962, p.

Bibliography

Adamiciewiez, A.: Die Blutgefasse des menschlichen rucken-
markes 1. Teil: Die Gefasse der ruchenmackssubstanz,
S. B. Heidelberg Acad. Wiss. 84:469–502, 1881. Ibid II
Teil: 85, 101–130, 1882.

Amato, V. P., and Bombelli, R.: Early skeletal and vascular
changes in rats fed on sweetpea (Lathykos odoratus)
seeds. J. Bone Joint Surg. [Br.] 41:600, 1959.

Anders, J. D.: Chromosome studies in scoliosis. *In* Proceedings of a Symposium on Scoliosis, held in London,
1965. P. A. Zorab (Ed.) London, 1965.

Anderson, H. B.: Anesthetic management of scoliosis
surgery. *In* Scoliosis, G. C. Robin (Ed.), Academic
Press, Inc., New York, 1973.

Badger, V. M.: Correlation studies on muscle in scoliosis;
histochemistry, electromyography, electromicros-
copy, and quantitative enzymes. J. Bone Joint Surg.
[Am.] 51:204, 1969.

Baker, J. P. (Ed.): Symposium on respiratory failure. Med.
Coll. Va. Q. 9:2, 1973.

Bates, D. V., Mackeems, P. T., and Christie, R. V.: Respiratory Function in Disease. W. B. Saunders, Philadelphia, 1971.

Beals, R. K.: Homocystinuria. A report of two cases and review of the literature. J. Bone Joint Surg. [Am.] 51-A; 1564, 1969.

Bergofsky, E. H., Turino, G. M., and Fishman, A. P.: Cardiorespiratory failure of kyphoscoliosis. Medicine [Balt.] 38:263, 1959.

Bisgard, J. D., and Musselman, M. M.: Scoliosis; its experimental production and growth correction; growth and fusion of vertebral bodies. Surg. Gynecol. Obstet. 70:1029, 1940.

Blount, W. P.: Bracing for scoliosis. *In* Orthotics, Etcetera, Physical Medicine Library, Vol. 9, Sidney Licht (Ed.), Elizabeth Licht, Publisher, New Haven, 1966.

Blount, W. P., and Bolinske, J.: Physical therapy in the nonoperative treatment of scoliosis. J. Phys. Ther. 47:10, 1966.

Brooks, L., et al.: The epidemiology of scolioses. A prospective study. J. Bone Joint Surg. [Am.] 55:436, 1973.

Chronic Obstructive Pulmonary Disease: A Manual for Physicians, ed. 3. National Tuberculosis and Respiratory Disease Association, New York, 1972.

Cochran, G. V. B., and Waugh, T. R.: The external forces in correction of idiopathic scoliosis. Proceedings of the Scoliosis Research Society. J. Bone Joint Surg. [Am.] 51:201, 1961.

Collis, D. K., and Ponseti, I. V.: Long-term followup of patients with idiopathic scoliosis not treated surgically. J. Bone Joint Surg. [Am.] 51:425, 1969.

Coner, P. E.: Histological study of tissues in scoliotic patients. J. Bone Joint Surg. [Am.] 53:199, 1971.

Cowell, H. R., Hall, J. N., and MacEwen, G. D.: Genetic aspects of idiopathic scoliosis. A Nicholas Andry Award essay. Clin. Orthop. 86:121, 1972.

DeGeorge, F. V. and Fisher, R. L.: Idiopathic scoliosis: Genetic and environmental aspects. J. Med. Genet. 4:251, 1967.

Dwyer, A. F., Newton, N. C., and Sherwood, A. A.: An anterior approach to scoliosis. A preliminary report. Clin. Orthop. 62:192, 1969.

Dwyer, A. F.: Anterior instrumentation for scoliosis. *In* Scoliosis, G. C. Robin (Ed.), Academic Press, Inc., New York, 1973.

Enneking, W. F., and Harrington, P.: Pathological changes in scoliosis. J. Bone Joint Surg. [Am.] 51:165, 1969.

Epstein, J. A., Epstein, B. S. and Lavine, L.: Nerve root compression associated with narrowing of the lumbar spinal canal. J. Neurol. Neurosurg. Psychiatry 25:165, 1962.

Epstein, J. A., Epstein, B. S., and Lavine, L. S.: Surgical treatment of nerve root compression caused by scoliosis of the lumbar spine. J. Neurosurg. 41:449, 1974.

Evarts, C. M., Winter, R. B., and Hall, J. E.: Vascular compression of the duodenum associated with the treatment of scoliosis: Review of the literature and report of eighteen cases. J. Bone Joint Surg. [Am.] 53:431, 1971.

Fried, L. C., and Doppman, J.: The Arterial Supply to the Lumbosacral Spinal Cord on the Monkey—a Comparison with Man. Personal Communication.

Galante, J., Schultz, A., Dewald, R. L., and Ray, R. D.: Forces acting in the Milwaukee brace in patients undergoing treatment for idiopathic scoliosis. J. Bone Joint Surg. [Am.] 52:498, 1970.

Glauber, A., Fernback, J. Massanyi, L., and Medgyesi, G.: Protein metabolism in idiopathic scoliosis. J. Bone Joint Surg. [Am.] 44:1553, 1962.

Gucker, T., III: Changes in vital capacity in scoliosis: Preliminary reports on effects of treatment. J. Bone Joint Surg. [Am.] 44:469, 1962.

Harris, E. D., Jr., and Sjoerdsma, A.: Collagen profile in various clinical conditions. Lancet. 2:707, 1966.

Harris, P.: Principles of management of cor pulmonale. Chest [Suppl. 2] 58:437–440, 1970.

Hirano, S.: Electron microscopic studies on back muscles in scoliosis. J. Jap. Ortho. Assn. 46:47, 1972.

Horae, J., Nachemson, A., and Scheller, S.: Clinical and radiological long-term follow-up of vertebral fractures in children. Acta Orthop. Scand. 43:49k, 1972.

James, J. I. P.: Scoliosis. Longman Inc., New York, 1968.

James, J. I. P.: Scoliosis. Pediatr. Clin. North Am. 1:225, 1967.

Kazmin, A. I., and Merkureva, R. V.: Biochemical study of the level of aminopolyglycons and glycoproteids in the spinal tissues of scoliotic patients. Ortop. Travmatol. Protez. 30:20, 1969.

Knutsson, F.: Vertebral geneses of idiopathic scoliosis in children. Acta. Radiol. [Diagn.] 4:395, 1966.

Langenskiold, A., and Michelsson, J. E.: The pathogenesis of experimental progressive scoliosis. Acta Orthop. Scand. [Suppl. 59] 1962.

Lin, H. Y., Nash, C. L., Herndon, C. H., and Anderson, N. B.: The effects of corrective surgery on pulmonary function in scoliosis. J. Bone Joint Surg. [Am.] 56:6, 1974.

Liszka, O.: Spinal cord mechanisms leading to scoliosis in animal experiments. Acta Med. Pol. 2:45, 1961.

MacEwen, G. G.: A look at the diagnosis and management of scoliosis (Ed.) Ortho. Rev. 3:9, 1974.

MacEwen, G. D., and Cowell, H. R.: Familial incidence of idiopathic scoliosis and its implication on patient treatment. J. Bone Joint Surg. [Am.] 92:405, 1970.

McKusick, V. A.: Heritable Disorders of Connective Tissue, ed. 4. C. V. Mosby Company, St. Louis, 1972.

Michelsson, J. E.: The development of spinal deformity in experimental scoliosis. Acta Orthop. Scand. [Suppl. 81], 1965.

Nachlas, I. W., and Borden, J. N.: The cure of experimental scoliosis by directed growth control. J. Bone Joint Surg. [Am.] 33:24, 1951.

Nash, C. L., Jr., and Moe, J. H.: A study of vertebral rotation. J. Bone Joint Surg. [Am.] 51:223, 1969.

Naeye, R. L.: Kyphoscoliosis and cor pulmonale. A study of the pulmonary vascular bed. Am. J. Pathol. 38:561, 1961.

Nordwall, A.: Studies in idiopathic scoliosis. Acta Orthop. Scand. [Suppl. 150], 1973.

Piggott, H.: Posterior rib resection in scoliosis. A preliminary report. J. Bone Joint Surg. [Br.] 53:663, 1971.

Ponseti, I. V.: Skeletal lesions produced by aminonitrites. Bull. Hosp. Joint Dis. 20:1, 1956.

Ponseti, I. V., Pedroni, V., and Dohrman, S.: Biochemical analyses of intervertebral discs in idiopathic scoliosis. J. Bone Joint Surg. [Am.] 54:1793, 1972.

Redford, J. B., Butterworth, T. R., and Clements, E. L., Jr.: Use of electromyography as a prognostic aid in the management of idiopathic scoliosis. Arch. Phys. Med. and Rehabil. 50:433, 1969.

Riseborough, E. J.: The effects of scoliotic deformities in pulmonary function. In Scoliosis, G. C. Robin (Ed.), Academic Press, Inc., New York, 1973.

Risser, J. C.: The iliac apophysis: An invaluable sign in the management of scoliosis. Clin. Orthop. 11:111, 1958.

Risser, J. C.: Scoliosis: Past and present. J. Bone Joint Surg. [Am.] 46:167, 1964.

Roaf, R.: The basic anatomy of scoliosis. J. Bone Joint Surg. [Br.] 480:786, 1966.

Samuelson, S.: Cor pulmonale resulting from deformities of the chest. Acta Med. Scand. 142:399, 1952.

Silverman, B. J., Graham, J. J.: Cast syndrome and scoliosis. Bull. Hosp. Joint Dis. 31:97, 1970.

Stearns, G., Chen, J. Y. T., McKinley, J. B., and Ponseti, I. V.: Metabolic studies of children with idiopathic scoliosis. J. Bone Joint Surg. [Am.] 37:1028, 1955.

Tureen, L. L.: Circulation of the spinal cord and the effect of vascular occlusion. Res. Publ. Assoc. Res. Nerv. Ment. Dis. 18:394, 1938.

117

Verbiest, H.: Neurogenic intermittent claudication in cases with absolute and relative stenosis of the lumbar vertebral canal and cases with narrow lumbar intervertebral foramina, and in cases with both entities. Clin. Neurosurg. 20:204, 1972.

Warner, T. F. C. S., Shorter, R. G., McIlrath, D. C., and Dupree, E. L.: The cast syndrome. J. Bone Joint Surg. [Am.] 56:1263, 1974.

Waters, R. L., and Morris, J. M.: An in vitro study of normal and scoliotic interspinous ligaments. J. Biomech. 6: 343, 1973.

Yoss, R. E.: Vascular supply of the spinal cord: The production of vascular syndrome. Univ. Mac. Med., Bull. 16:333, 1950.

Zaoussis, A. L., and James, J. I. P.: The iliac apophysis and the evaluation of curves in scoliosis. J. Bone Joint Surg. [Br.] 40:442, 1958.

Index

119

120

121